Time*less*

Time*less*

KARA DAVIS, MD

SILOAM

TIMELESS by Kara Davis, MD
Published by Siloam
Charisma Media/Charisma House Book Group
600 Rinehart Road
Lake Mary, Florida 32746
www.charismahouse.com

Visit the author's website at. www.DrKaraDavis.com.

Cover design by Lisa Rae McClure
Design Director: Justin Evans
Cover photography by Karen Forsythe,
www.karenforsythephotography.com

Library of Congress Cataloging-in-Publication Data:
Davis, Kara.
  Timeless : your mind, body, and spirit guide to aging with grace and
confidence / Kara Davis, MD. -- First edition.
      pages cm
  Includes bibliographical references.
  ISBN 978-1-62998-596-1 (trade paper) -- ISBN 978-1-62998-597-8
(e-book)
  1. Aging--Religious aspects--Christianity. I. Title.
  BV4580.D38 2015
  248.8'5--dc23
                          2015027624

While the author has made every effort to provide accurate Internet
addresses at the time of publication, neither the publisher nor the author
assumes any responsibility for errors or for changes that occur after
publication.

First edition

15 16 17 18 19 — 987654321
Printed in the United States of America

To my mother and mother-in-law,
Eura Foster and Phyllis Davis,
who epitomize aging with grace.
And in loving memory of my father,
Walter Thomas (1925–2014).

CONTENTS

Introduction

FIGHTING THE CLOCK

This is the day the LORD *has made; we*
will rejoice and be glad in it.

—PSALM 118:24, MEV

AMERICA IS GROWING older. Much older. In 2011 the number of people over sixty-five totaled 41.4 million. At the start of the "Baby Boomer" generation, the numbers of seniors only measured 10 million. Yet demographers project that by 2050 the elderly population will reach nearly 80 million.[1]

Not only are we reaching retirement age by the droves (some estimate ten thousand per day), we are living longer once we get there. The average sixty-five-year-old can expect to live about two more decades. This rapid change in our country's demographics has affected every aspect of our society. Health care and housing in particular are feeling the impact. To be sure, growing old and living long might *appear* to be simple matters, but they bring a myriad of complex issues to the table. And these are matters we cannot ignore. News programs feature interviews with respected economists, asking their projections of things to come. The prevailing question: "Are we ready?"

This is a valid question because preparation today is the key for tomorrow. Even now, local, state, and federal governments are preparing policies to help offset this huge demographic shift. While this is good, government strategies aside, let's admit there is more to the equation. We may face a national crisis. Yes, the *nation* is aging. But guess what? So am I. So are you. And so are our parents.

Although we all may recognize the impact this will have on the *country*, if we explore the fuller dimension, we must admit this brings a *personal* impact. As much as we may try to ignore it, every morning when we look into the bathroom mirror, our reflection says, "You aren't so young anymore."

And you know what? That's not so bad. By all means, we should be thankful for long life. I chose Psalm 118:24 to open this book because it's a great reminder of how each day is a gift from our heavenly Father. The passing years give us so many reasons to rejoice; longevity is indeed a blessing. To be sure, Psalm 118:24 issues a wonderful reminder of how we ought to feel. Yet another verse prior to this one speaks to the issue more candidly: "The days of our lives are seventy years; and if by reason of strength they are eighty years, yet their boast is only labor and sorrow; for it is soon cut off, and we fly away" (Ps. 90:10).

Moses, who wrote the latter psalm, sizes up aging well. Now don't get me wrong; no one can deny that long life is a blessing. But with each passing year come challenges we couldn't have imagined in our years of idyllic youth. After we have prevailed through obstacles, triumphed over hurdles, and against all odds endured the race—we die. Wow. Yes, Moses's assessment hits the target. In eloquent yet frank language, he hits the nail on the proverbial head.

So this book is about growing old (growing "older" might be a gentler term). I will shamelessly admit I wrote it with a personal agenda. For me, there was something about receiving my AARP (American Association of Retired Persons) card in the mail. This watershed moment hit me like a jolt of electricity. I held the envelope and stared. In that surreal instant the awareness hit: I'm *officially* "over the hill." In other words, the odds are high that my days remaining are fewer than those I've lived. Once again—Wow.

No question, aging changes everything. It sweeps into our lives—physically, mentally, interpersonally, and financially. It even reaches down to the mundane. Take skin care products, for instance. In my pre-AARP life, the choice of what I'd use to wash and moisturize my face was pretty simple. I bought whatever happened to be on sale. Not now. I invariably search for the key phrase: anti-aging. Even though those two little words are sure to hike the price, I feel peace. I'm OK with spending more money (sometimes, a whole lot more). Although frugal by nature, I've learned how to rationalize the cost:

- "I'm investing in myself."
- "You get what you pay for."
- "Why not, it's just money—and I'm *worth* it!"

It's hard to believe. I never imagined it would happen. I have officially jumped on the bandwagon. I'm part of the mass of people taking a stand against the clock.

All kidding aside, we know there is nothing that can stop the clock. While powerless to stop the passage of time, we maintain considerable control over *how* we age. Our goal, then, should be to optimize the effect that time has on our total being—the body, mind, and spirit. One of my purposes in writing this book is to help us discover there is much to gain with every passing year. So let's welcome each day, go with the flow, and age with grace.

I hope *Timeless: Your Body, Mind, and Spirit Guide* is helpful to you, whether you are still fairly young in your forties, or a nonagenarian who can declare with each page, "Been there, done that, got the T-shirt." I also pray this book inspires you with the many lessons I have gleaned from the men and women in the Scriptures. Indeed, the Bible is a treasured source of encouragement and hope, so don't let the words of Moses steal your joy. That is not the Lord's intent for Psalm 90! Make a habit of embracing each day—even the difficult ones—as a gift from God. Challenges notwithstanding, this is still the day the Lord has made—so rejoice!

Chapter 1

ADVANCE CARE PLANNING

For the living know that they will die...
—ECCLESIASTES 9:5, NIV

O NLY AFTER I decided to write a book on aging did I recognize the broadness of this topic. When it came time to
organize the book, I considered a few ways to arrange the
chapters, finally opting on alphabetical order. Previously, I didn't
realize that "advance care planning" would come first. Yet as a
foundational concept it is the best place to start, since so much falls
under the umbrella of advance care planning (ACP). But whether
the issue is medical, legal, or financial, the above words of Solomon
capture the gist. ACP brings us face-to-face with this reality. It compels us to lay aside our emotions and tackle the raw truth. Practi-
cality is in order, not apprehension or evasiveness. The latter causes
us to procrastinate or avoid the issue altogether. This is not beneficial to us, and not fair to our families or other potential caregivers.

Every state has laws promoting living wills and/or durable
powers of attorney for health care. At the federal level, the Patient
Self-Determination Act of 1990 requires all health care institutions
receiving funds from Medicare or Medicaid to provide information
on end-of-life care to their patients. The government implemented
these measures out of respect for an individual's right to self-determination, including the right to accept or reject various treatments.

The crux of ACP is communication. Ideally we communicate our
goals and values to those closest to us, and they incorporate them
into our present and future treatment plans. The time to do this is

now, when we still have full cognitive capacity. Such planning will prove vital if we ever lose that capacity. While they are far from perfect, ACPs offer advantages on numerous fronts. They help to ensure the care we receive toward the end of our lives is consistent with our preferences and that others respect our choices, even when we are no longer able to verbalize them. They also reduce the potential for conflict and guilt among family members, caretakers, and friends.

Given these advantages and the laws in place to promote their use, why is it that relatively few people (about 15 percent of adults) have created advance care plans? For some it's simple procrastination. Others might not understand the purpose, or they underestimate the benefits. Whatever the case, many people never address end-of-life matters, whether formally or informally. They don't spell out their preferences in a document or even communicate them to a loved one verbally. The final result is speculation over matters of extreme importance; this is not good.

For the sake of illustration, imagine this scenario. Along with your family, friends, and health care providers, you are invited to a dinner in your honor. The occasion offers a twist, though. The guests must decide what you will eat. Some are confident you would enjoy steak, while others insist you would choose seafood. A few folks think salad is best. However, you would *really like* a chicken sandwich, which is the one menu item everyone overlooked.

Since all the guests *know* you, they believe their choice *for* you matches what you would choose for yourself. Lively conversation escalates into an argument, with one person prevailing because of seniority, persuasion, or intimidation. Yet whatever means he or she uses to earn the right to decide, that person's decision will be incorrect. The wrong choice won't stem from carelessness or insensitivity, but from the fact that you never told anyone how much you like chicken sandwiches.

This speaks to values. Two people can be very close—even intimate—but it does not mean they embrace the same values. Couples can relate: what is significant to one might be irrelevant to the other. This is why ACPs are not just useful for health care providers, but especially beneficial to those we love. These plans release them from the burden of making decisions *for* us without having input *from* us. Ideally, they replace confusion and strife with peace and assurance. In our restaurant scenario, a quarrel ensued over a trivial matter. Imagine the potential for conflict if the decision is not about food, but how you spend your last days on this earth.

BIBLICAL INSIGHTS

> To everything there is a season, a time for every purpose under heaven: a time to be born, and a time to die.
> —ECCLESIASTES 3:1–2, MEV

The Bible says King Solomon was the wisest man who ever lived. The story appears in 1 Kings, when "the LORD appeared to Solomon in a dream by night; and God said, 'Ask! What shall I give you?'" (1 Kings 3:5). Solomon prayed for wisdom, specifically a heart of understanding and the capacity to discern right from wrong.

Solomon's writings are packed with pearls of wisdom. In Ecclesiastes, written in his later years, he delves into some of the more challenging issues about our life span and existence. While you won't find the term "advance care planning," the verses are filled with insights related to the topic, including the gem about time, seasons, and cycles. He starts the third chapter with two significant points in the life cycle—birth and death—and draws a parallel to the cycles of nature. Just as the seasons transition from one to the next, so do the stages of life. Each day has a dawning and a sunset. So does each life.

As such, planning for death should come as naturally as planning for the seasons to change. Consider how "no-nonsense" we are when it comes to preparing for winter. The need to replace screen windows with storm windows or winterize the car is hardly a touchy subject. We should be just as sensible with the fact that the "winter season" of life is inevitable. God doesn't hide this; He even reveals it in nature. Don't be paralyzed by fear. Rather, be practical and plan accordingly.

ACP ELEMENTS

Living wills

Advance care plans are just that—plans. There are many components to ACPs, including a "Living Will," also known as a "Health Care Declaration" or a "Health Care Directive." This is a document indicating what kinds of medical treatment, particularly life-sustaining measures, you *do* want or *do not* want. They include your preferences on such interventions as the following:

- Mechanical ventilation. This is also referred to as a being placed on a "breathing machine," "respirator," or "ventilator."

- Kidney dialysis. In severe illness, it is common for the kidneys to stop functioning properly. It is important to understand that dialysis does not *restore* kidney function, but *replaces* it. In some cases the kidneys recover their function and allow a suspension of dialysis, but in cases of permanent damage, treatment may continue indefinitely.

- Artificial nutrition and hydration. If your condition makes it impossible for you to eat and drink, nutrients and fluids can be given through an intravenous line or through a tube inserted into your stomach.

- Resuscitation. If the heart stops beating, resuscitation is used to maintain circulation. This is done by compressing the chest via cardiopulmonary resuscitation, or CPR, and/or by administering an electric shock to the chest, a process known as "cardioversion."

Do not resuscitate (DNR)

Directives on resuscitation are typically included in a living will but can also be written as a separate order. In other words, you can specify your desires for or against artificial resuscitation whether or not you have an ACP.

Artificial resuscitation usually includes more than just chest compressions and cardioversion. Intubation (where a flexible plastic tube is placed in the windpipe) and mechanical ventilation, as well as administration of heart-stimulating drugs, are all components. Some people, especially those with terminal illnesses or serious medical conditions, opt against any intervention in the event their heart stops beating. Such a choice means a "Do Not Resuscitate" (DNR) order must be written, placed in the medical record, and communicated to all health care providers. Additionally the various components of resuscitation can be spelled out in the order. For example, a person might be willing to undergo cardioversion or chest compressions but not to be placed on a ventilator.

Like all other features of an advance care plan, DNR orders are not "written in stone." Over the course of time, as life's circumstances change, it is not uncommon for an individual to modify these arrangements. In addition, DNR orders may need to be adjusted for specific circumstances. Some hospital policies, for instance, require the DNR order to be suspended during any surgical procedure requiring general anesthesia, and then reinstated after the operation. A DNR order is generally required to be eligible for hospice care. Laws vary from state to state, so check with your hospital administrator or health care provider for further information.

Issues and obstacles

One thing in life is certain—there's often a huge divide between theory and practice. Advance care plans prove the truth of this observation. While the concept makes good sense, there are many barriers to accomplishing their objectives. Some common ones include the following:

- *Ambiguous phrases.* The terminology used in living wills can be vague, using such subjective phrases as "heroic measures" or "imminent death." One person's idea of what constitutes "heroic" or "imminent" can vary widely from the next. So the potential for conflict still exists, even when there is a properly executed document.

- *Allowance for the unexpected.* What happens if the living will specifies no mechanical ventilation, but a person has an accident at a swimming pool and nearly drowns? Is it appropriate to withhold resuscitation in *all* scenarios, even if a full recovery is expected?

- *Prognostic uncertainty.* In most cases, prognosis can be measured with only a *reasonable* degree of certainty, not with *absolute* certainty. Even if the prognosis is entirely accurate, the length of time remaining—whether days, weeks, or months—is subject to the biases and values of the one interpreting the document.

For these and other reasons, many people will designate an individual to serve as their Health Care Proxy.

Health Care Proxy

Health Care Proxy statutes allow for the selection of a health care durable power of attorney. This is usually a family member or friend who assumes the role of a surrogate. They are legally authorized to act as the patient's representative for health care decisions. They are granted authority to make decisions when the patient has lost the capacity to do so, thereby reducing confusion in interpreting the living will.

BIBLICAL INSIGHTS

The wise man's eyes are in his head, but the fool walks in darkness. Yet I myself perceived that the same event happens to them all.
—ECCLESIASTES 2:14

One pervasive theme in Ecclesiastes is that no one is spared the contingencies of life. Regardless of intelligence, status and skills, all are subject to "time and chance" (see Ecclesiastes 9:11). This is why selecting a Health Care Proxy is a good idea. Though a difficult concept to accept, all of us will eventually lose our capacity to make decisions. This is inevitable, and happens in one of three ways: a decline in physical health, a decline in cognitive functions, or death. What we *don't* know is the when, why, and how—that unpredictable aspect of life Solomon describes so eloquently. As such, the ideal time for selecting such a proxy is as a young adult. Remember, should circumstances and relationships change, you can always change your selection as you grow older.

Keep in mind, the person who assumes this role is responsible for making decisions in your stead. Others will freely share their opinions, but your proxy has the final say. He or she is not just another voice in the "consensus choir"; this person assumes the role of "choir director." Health care providers look to the proxy for definitive answers. As such, it is important to select your surrogate wisely and communicate with this person regularly. If you do not name a proxy, state law designates a sequence of family members who will assume this role by default. Recognize, however, that the person identified by the state might not be the person you would choose.

Surrogate decisions follow three standards:

- Substituted judgment. The surrogate uses his or her knowledge of your past values and preferences to make decisions.

- Best interest. If a situation arises where it is impossible to figure out what you would want, the proxy makes a decision based on what a reasonable person would deem best.

- Clear and convincing. This is a much stricter standard which requires that the proxy have a solid knowledge of your preferences, either orally or written.

Always keep in mind the objective of advance care planning. The goal is to preserve the ideals and respect the desires of the person who can no longer make decisions. In that light, I'm reminded of biblical passages where Jesus made a distinction between the letter of the law and the spirit of the law. Life is full of the unexpected. In addition, options for medical care are not stagnant; they continuously evolve. It is entirely feasible for doctors to develop new therapies, new medications, and new approaches after you write your ACP. So situations may arise that would have been absolutely impossible to foresee. When that happens, your proxy must be willing to shift gears from strictly adhering to the letter of the ACP and instead embrace the spirit of it. The latter approach places the essence of your personality at the forefront rather than a cut-and-dried document. I am not minimizing the importance of the document—we all should have one. But it is a tool for guidance. It should not make us lose sight of what's important.

BIBLICAL INSIGHTS

The father of the righteous will greatly rejoice, and he who begets a wise child will delight in him. Let your father and your mother be glad, and let her who bore you rejoice.

—PROVERBS 23:24–25

Though Solomon wrote the vast majority of the Book of Proverbs, he is not the author of this particular verse or others found in later chapters. Still, as the book's compiler, his views are reflected in these proverbs, even those he didn't write. Certainly Solomon had much to say about the ups and downs of parenting. And he spoke from experience, considering he had "seven hundred wives, princesses, and three hundred concubines" (1 Kings 11:3). No telling how many kids he had!

As Solomon grew older, his heart turned away from God—no thanks to all those wives! But when he slipped into idolatry, did it impact his parenting skills? Possibly—although some of his children must have been born while he was devoted to God and blessed with supernatural wisdom. Unfortunately being a wise parent didn't guarantee that his children would turn out wise. Case in point: after he died, his son Rehoboam made a decision so stupid it ripped the kingdom in two! Indeed, when Solomon said, "A wise son makes a glad father, but a foolish son is the grief of his mother" (Prov. 10:1), he was speaking from the heart.

Keep in mind, even exceptional parents can give birth to what the Bible calls a "fool." And you wouldn't want a fool making weighty decisions on your behalf! This is why selecting a Health Care Proxy can become a real challenge, especially if you decide on someone other than your children. Be objective and prepared to make the tough choices, no matter how sticky.

Organ and tissue donation

Becoming an organ and tissue donor requires that you enroll in your state's donor registry. You should also communicate your request to your family and include it as part of your ACP. Misconceptions of organ donations abound, including the notion that older men and women are not qualified—as if our organs somehow pass their "expiration date." On the contrary, when it comes to organ donation, age is only a number. During the year 2012, 32 percent of donors were over age fifty. A team of transplant professionals makes the final decision about what tissues (if any) can be donated. Although a factor, age is not the only criteria. Currently about one hundred million people are registered in the United States. While that sounds like a large number, it falls short of need. Nearly twenty people die each day waiting for an organ.

That brings us back to the issue of misconceptions. Organs are assessed for transplant *after* a person is determined to be brain dead (the obvious exception is a living donation). Donors are often victims of accidents involving head trauma, or suffer brain damage suddenly from a stroke or ruptured cerebral aneurysm. But whatever the case, brain death has occurred. Why is this important? Because many people hold the erroneous belief that their organs might be removed before they are dead.

So what constitutes brain death? Meeting the following three criteria:

- Irreversible and unresponsive coma. Being comatose is not decisive, as some people in coma have a full recovery. The key terms are "irreversible" and "unresponsive," conditions that are determined by a clinical assessment.

- Absence of brain stem reflexes. Certain parts of the brain can be damaged, or even removed, without jeopardizing survival. Not so with the brain stem—its functions are life sustaining. There are several ways to assess this: Do the pupils of the eye react to bright light by constricting, or do they remain dilated? Do the eyes move when the head is turned? Is there any response to pain?

- Apnea, which refers to breathing, specifically the *absence* of respiration. In brain death, there are no spontaneous breaths taken once the ventilator is disconnected.

Thus, fears about organs being removed while someone remains alive are unfounded. In the United States it is illegal to sell organs, which provides another safeguard. At this time there is some discussion regarding the Dead Donor Rule, which governs the timing of organ removal. It is the standard currently followed in the United States, although other nations have less stringent criteria. A discussion of the pros and cons of the Dead Donor Rule is interesting, and highly charged, but beyond the scope of this book. I am a strong advocate of organ donation. It is a powerful, meaningful way to impact lives and pass on a blessing.

Hospice and palliative care

The word *hospice* is derived from the same Latin root as *hospitality* and *hospital*. It speaks to care, compassion, and accommodations. In the United States the hospice movement started in Connecticut in the mid-1970s. Now there are over three thousand organizations with steady growth. This is fueled, in part, by our aging population.

This term is used in several ways:

- *Hospice* refers to a *philosophy* of care that attends to the emotional, social, and spiritual needs, along with physical needs.

- *Hospice* is used to describe *organizations* providing end-of-life care.

- *Hospice* refers to the *location* where end-of-life care is received.

- *Hospice* denotes the specific *benefits* provided to Medicare Part A recipients.

In 1982 Congress approved the Medicare Hospice Benefit. Those with terminal illnesses are eligible to receive a wide range of services, including medical, nursing, social, and spiritual care. Medical equipment and supplies are covered, as well as physical, speech, and occupational therapy. Provisions to support caretakers and family members are available with home health services, housekeeping services, and bereavement support for up to one year after the death of the loved one.

Palliative care sets the foundation for hospice care. Some believe *palliation* is synonymous with *passivity*, but this is not so. It is *active* treatment provided to a person with a very serious disease. The primary goal shifts from "cure" to "comfort." While all hospice beneficiaries receive palliative care, the converse is not always the case. This is because a person may have an illness that fails to respond to available treatments (hence the need of palliative care) but still have a reasonable life expectancy. And it is life expectancy that determines hospice eligibility.

When curative therapy is unlikely, then the goal is to achieve the best quality of life possible for patients and families. Optimizing the quality of life is comprehensive and addresses physical, emotional, and spiritual needs. Comfort during the final stages of life requires adequate pain management, but also treatment for such things as depression, anxiety, and insomnia. The philosophy of hospice and palliative care is that the dying process is normal. The approach does not hasten death, but it does not postpone it either.

BIBLICAL INSIGHTS

Now King David was old, advanced in years; and they put covers on him, but he could not get warm. Therefore his servants said to him, "Let a young woman, a virgin, be sought for our lord the king, and let her stand before the king, and let her care for him; and let her lie in your bosom, that our lord the king may be warm." So they sought for a lovely young woman throughout all the territory of Israel, and found Abishag the Shunammite, and brought her to the king. The young woman was very lovely;

and she cared for the king, and served him; but the
king did not know her.
                                        —1 KINGS 1:1–4

I became a doctor before becoming a believer. Funny
how God arranged it so that I would approach the Bible
having a firmly established medical background. Initially, I found it intriguing. But years later my Old Testament professor, Dr. Robert L. Hubbard Jr., would help
me appreciate the concept of "preunderstanding" and
how it plays a major role in the way we study the Bible.

This passage is a case in point. Like many people, I
read it and chuckled over King David having a *thing*
for pretty women—which didn't fade with time! Obviously, his servants were aware of this penchant. They
made a point to find him someone "very lovely." But
because of my medical background (my "preunderstanding," as Dr. Hubbard would say), something else
about the passage was glaringly apparent. Long before
Medicare, the modern-day hospice movement, and the
incorporation of end-of-life studies in medical school
curricula, God provided an example of palliative care.

For all intents and purposes, Abishag was a hospice
nurse. She took care of the king and made his final days
as pleasant as possible. It appears theirs was an entirely
professional relationship. Notice that he didn't "know
her," meaning they weren't intimate. (And I don't believe
it was because he *couldn't* "know her"—see chapter 5 for
more on that discussion!) Interestingly his servants didn't
look for someone with a novel treatment or some new
drug. They weren't pursuing a cure. The end was near,
so they didn't seek to prolong the inevitable but to make
his remaining days comfortable. Even with measures as
simple as keeping the bed warm. I thank God for giving
us the story of Abishag, the prototype of palliative care.

People with terminal conditions and a life expectancy of six months
qualify for hospice care. Even though the majority have cancer, other

conditions like heart disease, lung disease, and neurological disorders (e.g., stroke, dementia, and Parkinson's disease) all qualify. The Medicare benefits allow for two initial ninety-day certification periods, followed by an unlimited number of sixty-day periods.

Even though hospice benefits provide for months and months of care, in 2000 the average stay was only twenty-five days, and 34 percent of deaths occurred within the first week of admission. Why the delay? Sometimes health care providers are not accurate in estimating life expectancy, or aren't familiar with the eligibility criteria. Sometimes patients are not ready to accept the prognosis, and their reluctance makes it easy for doctors to avoid the issue. "Sticky subjects" are hard to discuss, especially in the short time allowed for office visits.

However, at other times, health care providers just don't consider it. That has happened to me, especially when the terminal condition was not cancer. I once had a patient with complications from diabetes and hypertension. She had end-stage congestive heart failure and was frequently hospitalized. She and her daughters came to my office one day for a regular appointment, and before I could mention hospitalization, she said, "Dr. Davis, I'm tired." I knew what she was alluding to and felt an immediate sense of conviction over not enrolling her in hospice care much sooner. She and her daughters cried together while I made the arrangements for her to receive that care at home. Within a month she died comfortably in her own bed, surrounded by the people she loved.

About 70 percent of all deaths occur in a hospital, a long-term care facility, or in a nursing home. About half of all Americans die in an acute care hospital.[1] Anyone who has ever been there knows a hospital is not a place of calm and serenity, but lights, sound, frequent interruptions, and constant activity. If you have decided against resuscitation as part of your advance care plan, make sure you take time to discuss hospice with your family and health care provider. That way, enrollment will not be delayed. Keep in mind, if you have decided *against* DNR, then you are not eligible for hospice benefits.

Because the population is aging, we will likely see an expansion of hospice services and an even more pronounced focus on palliation. We now live in an era where people in their fifties, sixties, and seventies commonly have living parents. So hospice becomes a matter to consider from a personal standpoint (what we want for ourselves) as well as from the perspective of the aging parents. In September 2014, my father died after a long battle with prostate cancer. He never developed any signs of dementia but maintained full cognitive function until the very end. Consequently, he was keenly aware that his body was weakening and his strength declining. So he needed more than just *physical* palliation; he also needed comfort from an emotional and existential standpoint. My sisters and I were blessed to find a phenomenal hospice organization that sent us a team of "angels." Their mission: to make Dad's transition as comfortable as possible. And they succeeded. While I have always been a proponent of hospice care, previously this came from the perspective of a physician. Now I'm able to recommend it based on personal experience.

Final arrangements

No advance care plan is complete without a consideration of final arrangements. Let me share a personal story about my cousin, a practical man to the very end. When a doctor diagnosed him with cancer, he bought a calendar to keep track of everything—what I call the "package deal" of chronic illness. He managed a multitude of appointments with doctors, nurses, and care coordinators, being careful to reserve time to do things he enjoyed.

However, he didn't stop there. Along with his daily schedule, he planned his own funeral. Some will call this "morbid" and others will think it's "over the top." Before jumping to conclusions, consider some of the benefits.

BIBLICAL INSIGHTS

Let us hear the conclusion of the whole matter:
Fear God and keep His commandments, for this
is man's all.
—ECCLESIASTES 12:13

After reading the first few chapters of Ecclesiastes, the idea of planning your own funeral doesn't seem so far-fetched! The book paints a clear picture of the inevitable: we're born, we live, and we die. Indeed, the reader might be left wondering, "What's the point?" But Solomon's goal was not to leave us cynical. To the contrary, the book—when read in its entirety—strengthens our faith and gives hope to anyone questioning the meaning of life. By drawing on personal experiences, Solomon helps us avoid pitfalls that can lead to bitterness. His message is clear: status, wealth, and possessions don't make life significant. If we're not careful, such "things" can draw us into an existential void. While it is fine to set goals, we won't find long-term contentment and a sense of purpose by achieving them. Our primary pursuit ("man's all," according to this verse) must be God. Jesus put it this way: "But seek first the kingdom of God and His righteousness, and all these things shall be added to you" (Matt. 6:33).

So, to go back to my cousin's arranging his funeral, consider all the "to do's" involved:

- Drafting a budget

- Selecting a funeral director

- Choosing a location for the services (church, funeral home, residential)

- Deciding on ground burial, mausoleum, or cremation

- Finding a cemetery

- Purchasing a casket or urn
- Arranging the order of services (e.g., music, inspirational readings, the eulogist)
- Writing the obituary
- Newspaper announcements, floral arrangements, creating a memorial table or board
- Assigning pall bearers
- Provisions and location for a repast

Add to that a myriad of unexpected loose ends and then pile the responsibility on an emotionally distraught spouse, child, or relative. Seemingly mundane decisions turn complicated: Which photograph will go on the cover of the obituary? What songs? Who will sing them? Will resolutions be read, and if so, how many? To make matters worse, these "simple" decisions can generate serious conflict. So from a practical standpoint, anything that can be organized and paid for before your death will lighten the load for grieving family members and friends. Plus, they will have the assurance that you would be pleased with everything. After all, you put it together. It is not morbid, but a final act of kindness. My cousin's wife was extremely grateful that he loved her enough to do most of the work for her.

FAITH VS. FEAR

Some patients are unforgettable. Health care providers will agree there are people who, for whatever reason, become emblazoned in our memories. For me, one such patient was "Rhonda." She was in her fifties when she came to see me about a lump in her breast she detected several years earlier. Rhonda had been to several doctors, who all recommended surgery. However, she didn't think that was the right approach. Her casual demeanor threw me off guard. I expected to find a pea-sized lump. Instead, I found a tumor about the size of a baseball, and as hard as a rock. In one area it had broken through the skin, so she covered it with gauze to keep the drainage from staining her clothing. No question—it was cancer.

Rhonda hadn't had the tumor removed early on because her family believed she could be healed through prayer alone. She even declined my recommendation to see an oncologist. The only reason she made the appointment to see me? Someone told her I was a Christian, and she wanted me to join the circle of family and friends who were praying for her healing.

Over the course of the next year, the cancer took her life. For me, the worst part was not that she missed a window of opportunity for cure. The greater tragedy was how those close to her responded to her impending death. They believed the outcome reflected how firmly she believed in God's ability to heal. In other words, He could restore her physical body to a state of perfect health—provided she was convinced He could. They conveyed the message, *Rhonda, if you aren't healed, it's your own fault.*

During the last weeks of her life, Rhonda carried a heavy emotional burden: *she* was to blame for the cancer, *she* was the reason why a miracle had been denied, and *she* was responsible for her family's grief. This "theology" did not provide the sense of a compassionate God and a gentle Father. Rather, it left the impression that He made "empty promises." The chance to be healed was held out like a carrot on a string. She was the proverbial mule, working hard for what seemed to be within her grasp, only to find it was unreachable.

In this final section I will delve into the "gray zones" of end-of-life care, which makes for an appropriate way to close a chapter on advance care planning. As believers, at what point do we cross the line from "standing on the promises of God" to misinterpreting the Bible? How do we guard against superimposing our *personal* desires onto genuine faith? And how do we take on the attitude of Jesus—who said, "Nevertheless not My will, but Yours, be done" (Luke 22:42)—when faced with life-or-death situations? I'm obliged to include a disclaimer here: I'm not a theologian, and I have yet to earn a degree in religious studies. My perspectives come from my experiences as a physician, a student of the Bible, and an observer of life.

BIBLICAL INSIGHTS

You do not know what is the way of the wind, or how the bones grow in the womb of her who is with child, so you do not know the works of God who makes everything.
—ECCLESIASTES 11:5

As defined by the *Encarta Dictionary, trust* means "confidence in and reliance on good qualities, especially fairness, truth, honor, or ability." That is an apt description of how we respond to *people*. But trusting *God* takes on an added dimension. It requires that we never be leery about His actions. It is fair to be cautious when it comes to people; we have all likely known someone to be trustworthy who proved otherwise. Not so with God. His nature is honesty and integrity. His decisions are *always* correct. This level of trust is difficult to sustain when it comes to terminal illness and death. In times of pain and sorrow, we're prone to forget the truth found in Ecclesiastes 11:5, that we "do not know the works of God." So, like Job, we expect the impossible: we want an explanation that is rational, when our human minds don't have the capacity to understand all the ways of God. Yes, it's OK to ask why (after all, He's our loving Father). But genuine trust means we're still OK, even if He doesn't give an answer.

We all have an appointment with death. Unless we are alive when the Lord returns, we will one day transition through the process of physically dying. Yes, the Bible gives the story of Enoch and Elijah, who were "translated" into heaven and spared this experience. But there is no promise that any of us will be granted the same opportunity.

While the appointment is collective, the experience is unique. The timing and circumstances vary from person to person. Some die young; others die old. Some die comfortably; others die in pain. For some death is expected; it catches others by surprise. Some live recklessly but enjoy longevity, while others lead wholesome lives, yet die in their prime.

The thought of death stirs up a host of negative emotions such as fear, anxiety, isolation, or regret. Is God is able to heal? Of course He is. But all too often what motivates people to believe in a miraculous healing is fear. Rather than confront the fear governing their souls, they attempt to avoid the source of the fear, which is death. Since the only way to avoid death is through physical restoration, they cling to the possibility of healing and call it faith. This is not faith; it is an attempt to process toxic emotions like fear, anxiety, and regret. This causes confusion within the family, and can generate conflict between the family and the patient's health care team.

When a person has faith in Christ, such toxic emotions should not prevail. Negative feelings should be fleeting and quickly dispelled, never consume us. Why? Because of the advantages we have as believers. The apostle Paul, in his letters to the churches, makes the benefits clear:

- Death is not final: "For the wages of sin is death, but the gift of God is eternal life in Christ Jesus our Lord" (Rom. 6:23).

- Death ushers us into the presence of God: "So we are always confident, knowing that while we are at home in the body we are absent from the Lord. For we walk by faith, not by sight. We are confident, yes, well pleased rather to be absent from the body and to be present with the Lord" (2 Cor. 5:6–8).

- Death is not the winner: "So when this corruptible has put on incorruption, and this mortal has put on immortality, then shall be brought to pass the saying that is written: 'Death is swallowed up in victory. O Death, where is your sting? O Hades, where is your victory?'" (1 Cor. 15:54–55).

- Death doesn't leave us hopeless: "But I do not want you to be ignorant, brethren, concerning those who have fallen asleep, lest you sorrow as others who have no hope" (1 Thess. 4:13).

- Death leads to transformation: "For our citizenship is in heaven, from which we also eagerly wait for the Savior, the Lord Jesus Christ, who will transform our lowly body that it may be conformed to His glorious body, according to the working by which He is able even to subdue all things to Himself" (Phil. 3:20–21).

Of course, these promises don't nullify the normal desire for life. While our experience after death will be glorious, our human nature has a yearning to live and not die, even in the face of pain and affliction. Paul describes this paradox eloquently:

> For to me, to live is Christ, and to die is gain. But if I live on in the flesh, this will mean fruit from my labor; yet what I shall choose I cannot tell. For I am hard-pressed between the two, having a desire to depart and be with Christ, which is far better. Nevertheless to remain in the flesh is more needful for you.
> —Philippians 1:21–24

Interestingly the end-of-life challenges confronting us today weren't even a topic for discussion a few generations ago. Advances in science and technology have allowed us to cure diseases that were once uniformly fatal. Some seniors can recall when illnesses we now consider inconsequential posed major health threats. However, progress has opened the doors to ambiguity. At what point do we go from sustaining life to prolonging death? And when, if ever, do we stop intervening to let a disease take its natural course?

Unfortunately there are no clear-cut answers. End-of-life care is not "cookie cutter" medicine; each person's experience is unique. Still, I have observed a common thread. The state of the heart makes a world of difference. It determines whether a person makes difficult choices in a peaceful frame of mind or in a state of panic and uncertainty. Proverbs 4:23 advises, "Keep your heart with all diligence, for out of it spring the issues of life." Most certainly we should guard our hearts against the fear of death. Fear has an adverse effect on our capacity to make decisions (the "sound mind" spoken of in 2 Timothy 1:7). Where there is fear, anxiety, and regret you will also find the appeal to sustain life at any cost—even when it's futile.

On the other hand, if we dispel negative emotions with biblical truths, then those fork-in-the-road decisions won't trouble our souls. With a calm mind, we assess matters clearly. If we are not afraid to die, then we're able to evaluate treatment options objectively and accept or decline them rationally. We're less likely to pursue treatments that are futile or inappropriate. Likewise, when our earthly relationships have been typified by love and forgiveness, then approaching the end is less troubling.

Every now and then I come across articles featuring "pearls of wisdom" from men and women in the winter season of life. They give guidance on what, if anything, they would do differently if they had the chance to start life over again. Some of the tips are pretty lightweight—take up a new hobby, travel the world, or master a skill. But others are more serious. And these are the gems that can dispel fear and facilitate peace as the days of living wind to a close. Invariably, three recurrent themes emerge relating to how we spend our time, the quality of our relationships, and where we place our values:

- *Time.* Reserve time to build relationships. Spend time doing things you enjoy. Don't waste time worrying.

Spend time helping others. Understand that family and friends may cherish your time more than tangible gifts.

- *Relationships.* Show appreciation and always say "thank you." Don't hold a grudge. Be quick to forgive. Pursue reconciliation. Don't take people for granted. Say "I love you" often.

- *Values.* Don't spend all your energy trying to make money. Avoid placing too much emphasis on career advancement. Don't treasure the things that "moth and rust destroy and where thieves break in and steal" (Matt. 6:19).

Ideally a believer should spend his or her final days in peace. This is a time to reflect on God's grace and joyfully anticipate an eternity spent with Him. However, you won't achieve this frame of mind on your death bed. Peace at the *end* of life is something that is established *throughout* life. Ask yourself, "Which would I prefer for myself and my family—serenity or emotional turmoil?" Of course, we would all choose the former. But the assurance of a peaceful end is sealed during the days of life, by way of daily decisions. It comes through making wise choices with respect to time, relationships, and values. It comes by choosing a path that minimizes regret and diminishes fear. This is what I call *authentic* advance care planning. Of course we should make sure we iron out the medical and legal details. Yes, we should communicate the specifics to our families and health care providers. However, don't forsake what is most important. In the end, how you live each day is what makes the difference.

Chapter 2

ATTITUDES AND EMOTIONS

*A person's wisdom brightens their face
and changes its hard appearance.*

—ECCLESIASTES 8:1, NIV

C HICAGO'S MUSEUM OF Science and Industry has a fascinating display on longevity. This creative, interactive exhibit provides the visitor with a wealth of knowledge on what lengthens (and shortens) our years. Naturally, what we eat and drink, the environment, our habits, and our DNA all play key roles. However, an often-overlooked component of long life is not related to the physical body. Longevity is also determined by what goes on in our minds. The part of the museum's exhibit that speaks to this draws a huge crowd—at least every time I have visited. It is a wall of faces of men and women who lived into their nineties and hundreds. The exhibit includes biographical sketches with descriptions of how major events and the social climate of the past century affected them and their families. I love putting on a headset and pushing a button to listen to these nonagenarians and centenarians give suggestions on what they believe prolongs life.

While their advice varies, it contains a few recurrent themes. I'm not surprised that a nutritious diet and exercise are high on each of their lists. Yet all have something to say about the role of attitude and feelings. In particular, they emphasize the importance of freeing the mind from negative thoughts and emotions. None of them held grudges, they weren't prone to worry, and they made a habit of looking on the bright side. From their perspective (and I consider them all to be "experts" on living), longevity depends as much on mental and emotional well-being as it does physical health.

What especially intrigues me is something the museum didn't mention: all of their pleasant facial expressions. These men and women had survived serious hardships, such as war, poverty, the effects of Jim Crow segregation, and the Great Depression. Despite the lack of "easy living," they retained a lovely countenance. Decades of emotions left indelible marks on their faces. Their wrinkle lines confirmed that through the years, they smiled more than they frowned and laughed more than they cried. This is what the opening verse speaks to: conditions on the *inside* will show up on the *outside*. In this chapter I will address aging gracefully from the perspective of the mind. Our goal is to optimize our total well-being, which includes our emotions, our attitudes, and our mental health.

Attitudes and Emotions

Forgiving vs. bitterness

The need to forgive is not age specific. It is God's expectation for young and old alike. The difference between the two age extremes is that passing time brings with it more opportunities for offense. If we don't practice forgiveness while we are young, we will find ourselves consumed by its consequences when we age—and there are serious consequences that come from holding a grudge.

As an analogy, think about weeds. The best *time* to deal with a weed is when it first appears. The best *way* to deal with it is by pulling it up from the roots. When the beautiful green lawn of our soul is offended, an ugly weed appears. If we diligently inspect the lawn and pull the weed the instant it sprouts, we will restore its beauty right away. But woe to us if we fail to inspect, and double woe if we fail to pull! It doesn't take long for the tender root of the young plant to grow thick, deep, and gnarly. At the same time, brand new offenses (an unavoidable part of life) continue to dot our lawn with more and more weeds. Over time the lush landscape becomes a field of weeds and the kindness of youth turns bitter with age.

You don't have to be a Bible scholar to know God expects us to forgive. Consider this: the model prayer of Jesus (also called "The Lord's Prayer") includes a line about forgiveness: "And forgive us our debts, as we forgive our debtors" (Matt. 6:12). I memorized this prayer long before I became a believer; you may have as well. If not, I still believe we have the intrinsic awareness that we *should* forgive. However, our natural human tendency is to hold a grudge. We will even rehearse the offense in our minds, and share the details with others (which opens the door to gossip, another trait that takes the grace out of aging).

This is why it's so important to understand the nature of forgiveness. It is not based on emotions. Rather, it is a decision of the heart. We can't wait until we *feel* like forgiving. We must *choose* to forgive and let our feelings follow suit. Over the years, as a physician and pastor's wife, I have counseled with numerous people who fail to grasp this concept. So instead of subjecting their feelings, they nurture the hurt. Justifying and rationalizing their refusal to forgive, they keep the wounds fresh. It's as if they decide, "So what if the weeds take root? Who cares if my lawn is destroyed?" God cares.

Clinging to bitterness and denying forgiveness has consequences, especially in the physical realm. Some ailments more common with age may represent the manifestation of years of harboring resentments. I see this in my clinical practice, and the Bible affirms this reality. In Matthew 18, Peter asks Jesus how often he should forgive, and Jesus responds with a parable about a servant who owed a debt so great he couldn't possibly pay it. His master issued a punishment, but when the servant pleaded for mercy, the master had compassion and forgave the debt. Ironically, the same servant then showed no mercy to another man who owed him a much smaller sum of money. The unforgiving servant even threw the guy into prison. He would not forgive, though he had been forgiven.

Note the consequences. His master rebuked him and delivered a severe punishment: "And his master was angry, and delivered him to the torturers until he should pay all that was due to him" (Matt. 18:34). How much did this unforgiving servant owe? Consider that his lifetime earnings never would have resolved his debt. The master simply expected this servant to forgive just as he had been forgiven. When the wicked servant refused, he received a severe chastening. Until he was willing to forgive, he would be fair game for "the torturers."

Likewise, unless we forgive, we too can expect chastening. This is the point of parables, to give us lessons to apply to our lives. Because God is merciful, He does not sentence us to death—our eternal salvation is not in jeopardy. Still, we will face punishment for our hardened hearts. How might this chastening manifest itself in our lives? I believe one way is through physical affliction. Could it be that some of the burdens we attribute to "old age" may have their roots in an unforgiving heart? Might some of our ailments be evidence of "the torturers" Jesus spoke of in this parable? Scientific studies show that people who hold on to resentment, anger, and other toxic emotions are at greater risk for physical disease. Those who don't hold grudges tend to live longer, healthier lives. Now undoubtedly, the primary reason we should forgive is because we love God and obey His precepts. Still, if by chance you need additional motivation, try practicing forgiveness for the sake of your health.

Generosity vs. selfishness

In his apocryphal tale *A Christmas Carol*, Charles Dickens paints such a clear picture of Ebenezer Scrooge that the word "scrooge" appears in the dictionary—defined as "a miserly person." The story is set at Christmas Eve when Scrooge is an old man. But Dickens gives readers a glimpse into Scrooge's entire life, revealing that he was not always selfish. Though he had a knack for numbers and a frugal nature, he wasn't born miserly. So what happened? Scrooge never processed the painful experiences of his youth, and heartache hardened him. This, combined with the character flaw of greed, transformed his positive attribute of frugality into stinginess. Not only was he stingy; he was mean. (The two usually go hand in hand, with age strengthening the bond.)

One reason Dickens is considered a master storyteller is that his characters are so real. We can all relate to Scrooge because chances are, we know a couple. They might be relatives, neighbors, or friends. In fact, if we're honest, some of us are on our way to becoming Scrooge ourselves! Without question, misers don't grow old very well, because generosity is a key component to graceful aging.

BIBLICAL INSIGHTS

> Now there was one, Anna, a prophetess, the daughter of Phanuel, of the tribe of Asher. She was of a great age, and had lived with a husband seven years from her virginity; and this woman was a widow of about eighty-four years, who did not depart from the temple, but served God with fastings and prayers night and day. And coming in that instant she gave thanks to the Lord, and spoke of Him to all those who looked for redemption in Jerusalem.
>
> —LUKE 2:36–38

As an elderly widow, Anna likely didn't possess great wealth. Nevertheless, when it came to blessings and favor, she was extremely rich! Anna was a teacher of the Old Testament, one of only a few women mentioned in the Bible with this gift. She came from the tribe of Asher, not the priestly tribe of Levi. However, despite her gender and tribal heritage, she was well respected, even given a place to live on the temple grounds. Why so highly esteemed? Anna had a sacrificial spirit, giving her whole life to serving God. That is generosity in action.

Rest assured, her life wasn't trouble free. She spent the majority of her days a widow—her husband died after only seven years of marriage. While such painful circumstances might have hardened her heart, Anna

> let benevolence prevail. While she could have become a bitter old widow, she chose to live selflessly. And this selflessness led to exaltation, to the extent that her story is part of Scripture, written for all eternity. Anna personifies graceful aging. Her life bears witness to Proverbs 11:25: "The generous soul will be made rich."

If generosity leads to blessing, then why are so many people selfish? And why does this trait seem to become more common with age? I see several factors:

- The fear some have of others taking advantage of them. In many respects, generosity is a state of vulnerability and carries with it the risk of being "burned." Once burned, some will shield themselves at any cost—even at the cost of becoming a miser. In addition, past experience will affect present behavior. When people lose money for whatever reason, a tight fist is a common reaction. In the economic crisis of 2008, people lost huge sums of money; it cost some their life's savings. Not surprisingly, the level of charitable giving dropped precipitously during that period.

- There is the issue of trust. Some people are misers because they have no faith. They won't give because they don't believe God's promises, or they don't think He is able to replenish their bank account—and certainly not increase it!—if they give money away.

- Others simply allow greed and a tendency to hoard govern their lives.

While there are many reasons for selfishness, none are justifiable. True love is manifested in generosity. One of the most widely known verses in the Bible gives proof of this: "For God so loved the world that He gave His only begotten Son..." (John 3:16, emphasis added). Loving and giving are tightly linked. Love is the condition; generosity is the action. Examine the condition of your heart. Purge it of selfishness, and let generosity prevail.

Optimism vs. pessimism

Attitude is everything, especially when it comes to aging gracefully. Solomon speaks to the power of a positive outlook in several of his proverbs, including this one: "All the days of the afflicted are evil, but he who is of a merry heart has a continual feast" (Prov. 15:15). A cheerful disposition reveals itself on the face (recall the wrinkle lines from the museum exhibit). And research confirms that attitude—whether optimistic or pessimistic—has a tremendous impact on quality of life, physical well-being, and longevity.

Studies prove attitude influences even pain and functional capacity. One showed that two years following knee replacement surgery, pessimistic people had less improvement in knee function and significantly more pain, compared to optimistic people.[1] In conditions that cause chronic pain, pessimistic people are likely to focus on how they feel and slip into a mind-set of helplessness. When compared to optimists with the same degree of discomfort, pessimists tend to have higher levels of substances causing inflammation circulating in their bloodstreams. These chemicals *increase* sensitivity to pain. So attitude, in many respects, can have an analgesic effect.

Attitude has an especially strong impact on heart disease, the leading cause of death in the United States. In the Women's Health Initiative, a landmark project launched in 1991, investigators tracked nearly 162,000 women for more than fifteen years. At the start of the project, participants completed a questionnaire assessing several variables, including attitude. The researchers found that optimistic women had much lower rates of heart disease in comparison to pessimistic women. Interestingly, they discovered the same pattern when they evaluated the rate of death from all causes. Compared to optimists, pessimistic women were more likely to die from *anything*, not just heart disease.

Optimistic people have a faster rate of recovery after coronary artery bypass surgery and are able to return to normal activities sooner than pessimists. Compared to optimists, pessimists were found to be more likely to be readmitted to the hospital for such things as wound infections, angina, heart attack, or even the need to have a second bypass operation. And optimists had a better quality of life when measured six months after their operations.

Pessimism has a definite impact on longevity. In one study, the Mayo Clinic enrolled more than seven thousand people in the early 1960s and followed them for forty years. They found that people with pessimistic, anxious, and depressive personality traits had a higher rate of death, no matter what the cause. In another study conducted over a span of thirty years, researchers found that people who interpreted life's events in a pessimistic way had a 19 percent increased risk of mortality.

Finally in a project involving five hundred elderly men and women, participants were classified as having a "positive life orientation" if they answered "yes" to the following questions:

- Are you satisfied with life?

- Do you have a zest for life?

- Do you have plans for the future?

- Do you feel needed?

- Do you seldom feel lonely or depressed?

After a decade, of the 20 percent of participants classified as having a positive life orientation, nearly 55 percent were still alive, compared to 39 percent of those with a less-than-positive orientation. Interestingly, a positive attitude seemed to protect these individuals against the need for skilled nursing or other institutional care. After five years only about 3 percent of positive responders resided in nursing homes, compared with 18 percent of the rest.[2] So when it comes to aging—whether gracefully, energetically, or independently—attitude is everything!

Prejudice vs. love

Life is a learning experience. Ideally what we learn through the passing years should make us better people. This is the principle behind that simple expression, "If you knew better, you would do better." Surely there are many attributes of youth we are glad to leave behind, things we did because we didn't know any better. But there are several attributes of childhood we tend to forsake over time, when we ought to embrace them throughout our lives. Some of these relate to how we interact with other people, particularly people who are different from us. Children tend to be objective and impartial in their assessments, while adults "learn" intolerance, bias, and bigotry.

BIBLICAL INSIGHTS

The following day Jesus wanted to go to Galilee, and He found Philip and said to him, "Follow Me." Now Philip was from Bethsaida, the city of Andrew and Peter. Philip found Nathanael and said to him, "We have found Him of whom Moses in the law, and also the prophets, wrote—Jesus of Nazareth, the son of Joseph." And Nathanael said to him, "Can anything good come out of Nazareth?"

—JOHN 1:43–46

The Bible teaches through precept and example, providing plain and simple instructions. For example, those in the Ten Commandments like "Thou shalt not steal" or "Thou shalt not murder" are pretty clear cut. And while we won't find a specific scripture saying, "Thou shalt not embrace stereotypes," we are nevertheless taught this principle through examples like Nathanael.

We don't know much about this disciple—not nearly as much as we know about others like Peter, John, Thomas, and even Judas. Still, while limited in our glimpse of Nathanael, there is no reason to suspect he was a bad person. We can assume he was a good person—albeit with a character flaw. A flaw we shouldn't ignore. Indeed, since it is so common, we should learn from it.

Nathanael embraced a lie, even when he had a reason to reject it. Philip told him the Messiah had come, but rather than rejoice in this good news, Nathanael allowed his biased views to tarnish his response. His initial reaction to Jesus was negative only because he had preconceived (and erroneous) notions about Nazareth. Surely he was not *born* disliking Nazareth, but learned prejudiced views about the city as he grew older. To be sure, this character flaw is the foundation of many societal ills we see today. Do a little soul searching, and purge the flaw of prejudice if it rests in you.

One time a lawyer approached Jesus. Although a well-respected, highly educated man, he, like most Jews of that era, did not embrace people of different races and cultures. And he felt justified in his stance—he even thought God would agree with his biased views. He posed a question to Jesus, asking Him what he should do to inherit eternal life. After the Lord asked how he read the law, the lawyer posed another question in order to validate himself: "Who is my neighbor?" In response Jesus told the parable of the Good Samaritan (Luke 10:25–37), the rescuer from the despised race and the only one who helped a Jewish man victimized by thieves. In this story Jesus gave a lesson on humanity—love, mercy, and compassion are color blind. These Christlike virtues should never wane, but ought to become more evident in our lives over time.

Gratitude vs. thankfulness

Paul writes, "Rejoice always, pray without ceasing, in everything give thanks; for this is the will of God in Christ Jesus for you" (1 Thess.

5:16–18). We cannot overlook the glaring truth of these verses: *gratitude is not conditional!* If it were, then Paul would have said, "In good times, give thanks." Instead, he said "in everything." At all times and in all circumstances we have a reason to be grateful. This concept can present quite a challenge, especially as we grow older. Each passing year brings with it a measure of adversity. So how is it possible to feel appreciation in times of overwhelming trials and tribulation? How does one say "thank you" when confronted with illness, disability, financial hardship, or lost relationships?

It is not only possible; it is expected. How? First recognize that gratitude is not an emotion, but a condition of the heart. Certainly, in good times we feel a heightened sense of thanksgiving, but it does not follow that bad times should corrupt our hearts. The second step is to look at the big picture. Life's circumstances are always temporary, but God's grace toward us is eternal. If we focus on the big picture of grace, then gratitude naturally follows.

BIBLICAL INSIGHTS

And the LORD God prepared a plant and made it come up over Jonah, that it might be shade for his head to deliver him from his misery. So Jonah was very grateful for the plant.

—JONAH 4:6

When we consider the story of the prophet Jonah, what typically comes to mind is a lesson on obedience; namely, when Jonah defied God's command, he wound up in the belly of a fish. Yet the story yields several other teaching points, including gratitude. After Jonah preached God's message, the people of Nineveh repented. As a result, God showed mercy to them. Since Jonah despised them, this made him so angry that he even asked God to take his life.

The Lord taught His enraged prophet in a kind manner by using a real-life lesson. First He created a plant to give Jonah comfort from the sun and heat. As Jonah 4:6 indicates, Jonah responded with gratitude.

However, God then destroyed the plant and stirred up wind and heat so intense that Jonah grew faint. Attitude morphed into anger. When God challenged him, Jonah remained defiant. God then gently pointed out his irrational behavior: "But the LORD said, 'You have had pity on the plant for which you have not labored, nor made it grow, which came up in a night and perished in a night. And should I not pity Nineveh...?'" (Jon. 4:10–11).

When it comes to gratitude, the plant gave evidence of God's grace and unmerited favor. Jonah received kindness, though he didn't deserve it, especially after travelling in the opposite direction of where God told him to go. While momentarily pleased, Jonah didn't let that instant of gratitude transform his heart. If he had, the strong wind and sweltering heat would have made him more appreciative of God's kindness. He would have recognized that the Ninevites did not deserve God's grace—and neither did he! For Jonah, gratitude was just an emotion—stirred up by pleasant conditions, and disappearing rapidly when things got rough. Don't follow his example! Gratitude is more than a feeling; it is a condition of the heart.

Like forgiveness, gratitude is a decision, not a feeling. It is a conscious choice to keep our minds focused on what we have, not on what we don't have. There is a natural tendency to pay more attention to everything we are missing, especially if others in our circles enjoy those things. If we are not careful to guard our thoughts, a sense of entitlement (even envy) can supplant an attitude of gratitude. A heart of thanksgiving comes when we intentionally, and constantly, subject our minds to the Word of God: "Finally, brethren, whatever things are true, whatever things are noble, whatever things are just, whatever things are pure, whatever things are lovely, whatever things are of good report, if there is any virtue and if there is anything praiseworthy—meditate on these things" (Phil.

4:8). Through the power of the Holy Spirit, we have the capacity to control our thoughts. Keeping the mind focused on God—who He is and His bountiful blessings—will produce a grateful heart.

Contentment vs. complaining

Nobody wants to grow up to be a "grumpy old man" or a "grumpy old woman." Yet it happens all the time. When friends and family use phrases like, "She used to be so sweet and kind" to describe you, then rest assured, you've arrived. This doesn't happen overnight; it is a slow transition. Over the years your criticisms and complaints increase in frequency. This tendency may well be part of your personality. However, the character flaw often suppressed in youth comes out with a vengeance in old age. Seniority brings with it a sense of entitlement—many believe they've "earned" the right to complain.

Of course, this is not the case. The Bible clearly describes the desired quality of our speech: "Let no corrupt word proceed out of your mouth, but what is good for necessary edification, that it may impart grace to the hearers" (Eph. 4:29); and "Let your speech always be with grace, seasoned with salt, that you may know how you ought to answer each one" (Col. 4:6). Complaining does not line up with these commands. In addition to these *instructions*, God provides a good *example* in the Book of Exodus of how He feels about constant grumblers. After their miraculous deliverance from Egypt, the Israelites murmured and protested incessantly. For them, nothing was right about the wilderness—not the food, not the water, not Moses. God heard them and dealt with them accordingly. None of those whiners entered the Promised Land.

BIBLICAL INSIGHTS

Then Miriam and Aaron spoke against Moses because of the Ethiopian woman whom he had married; for he had married an Ethiopian woman. So they said, "Has the LORD indeed spoken only

> through Moses? Has He not spoken through us
> also?" And the LORD heard it.
>
> —NUMBERS 12:1–2

In many respects Miriam typifies the personality of the Israelites delivered from Egypt. When things were going well, the older sister of Moses celebrated God and worshipped Him through song and praise (see Exodus 15:20–21). When things weren't going so well, her celebration ceased. She swapped rejoicing for whining and encouragement for complaints. Here we see her epitomize an attribute of discontented people: anything and everything is fair game for criticism! In this passage the Israelites were in the middle of the wilderness, on their journey to the Promised Land. Of all the pressing issues at hand and the ways she could have assisted Moses, Miriam vented her hang-ups about her sister-in-law. Now, what did that have to do with anything? How was that any of Miriam's business? Yet a critical spirit often breeds illogical thinking.

Consider her thought process. How does it follow that, since Moses chose an Ethiopian wife, then God must have appointed her to lead the people too? And since she was older than Moses, at this time Miriam could have been in her nineties. What happened to the resourceful, clever young girl who took great risks to ensure her brother's safety? Something changed. Once a blessing to Moses, now Miriam represented a thorn in his flesh. After this episode, God caused leprosy to come upon her. The gracious prayer of Moses healed her, but she still died in the wilderness. Because of her grumbling, complaining, and discontent, Miriam never saw the Promised Land. Her life emphasizes the importance of Paul's words: "I have learned in whatever state I am, to be content" (Phil. 4:11).

The root of complaining is discontentment. And discontentment, according to Hebrews 13:5, is closely linked to coveting: "Let your conduct be without covetousness; be content with such things as you have. For He Himself has said, 'I will never leave you nor forsake you.'" When we covet, we long for what other people have, and become dissatisfied with what we have. While blinded to God's gracious provision, we somehow maintain 20/20 vision for all the things we're missing. This sets the stage for criticism, which fuels complaints. In the wilderness, the people rejected the miraculous food called manna. They expressed longing for the foods of Egypt, conveniently overlooking the fact that Egypt was the place of their enslavement. Ironically, during the wilderness period God addressed this tendency—even put it in writing. The last of the Ten Commandments says, "Thou shalt not covet" (Exod. 20:17, KJV).

For some, over time the tendency to be nitpicky and critical becomes second nature. Examine your speech. If you are fitting the bill for a grumpy old man or grumpy old woman, then purpose to change. Our speech reflects the state of our hearts. And when the heart is content, the complaining ceases.

Gentle vs. angry

To be sure, anger is not always destructive. Throughout the Bible, God manifests anger in response to injustice and wickedness. Through His example we learn that complacency is not the appropriate response to unfairness and oppression. God's display of righteous indignation sets an example for us to follow. For instance, racism and other societal ills should rouse us to action. As we mature, we should show godly anger more frequently and ungodly anger less frequently. Seniors cannot remain silent in the face of injustice and oppression. All too often we leave this fight to younger people, who may lack the influence, resources, and wisdom we older folks have at our disposal.

However, there is another form of anger that is anything but constructive. Righteous indignation is a virtue, but there is no place for anger grown from bitter roots. This is the anger we feel when we are offended; it is the kind that stirs a desire for revenge. Everyone has experienced it at some point, although the degree varies from person to person. Some exhibit anger as a personality trait and fume constantly. Irate by nature, when someone says, "Have a good day," they are likely to respond, "What's so good about it?" Others show sporadic anger, usually triggered by a personal offense. Both forms are toxic. If left unchecked, anger can lead to physical disease, particularly heart disease. And this risk only increases with time. So years spent harboring anger will make one mean, unpleasant—and ill.

BIBLICAL INSIGHTS

Then Naaman went with his horses and chariot, and he stood at the door of Elisha's house. And Elisha sent a messenger to him, saying, "Go and wash in the Jordan seven times, and your flesh shall be restored to you, and you shall be clean." But Naaman became furious...
—2 KINGS 5:9–11

While a courageous man of valor, Naaman faced a serious problem: he had leprosy. Yet the above passage identifies a more serious problem—anger management. So serious it nearly kept him from being healed of leprosy. After learning Elisha could help him, Naaman set out to find the prophet, traveling with the entourage of horses and chariots that went with high military rank. Naaman arrived at Elisha's house with pomp and circumstance, but this clearly did not impress the prophet. Elisha never came outside to greet him, instead sending a messenger with instructions on where Naaman should go and what he should do in order to be healed. Naaman responded with anger.

Naaman's rage stemmed from his unjustifiable sense of entitlement. His arrogance caused him to decide beforehand what represented suitable treatment for a man of his stature. And once he arrived, he deemed neither Elisha's behavior nor his advice acceptable.

Although Elisha's prescription held the key to his healing, it did not meet with his pride-driven standard. Naaman grew angry because what he *thought* he deserved did not come to pass. Funny how age can bring with it the same sense of entitlement. We can get irritated with friends and family members—not because of any specific offense—over similar feelings of privilege and prerogative. Like Naaman, we can place pride-driven expectations on those who, ironically, have our best interests at heart. In pique, we lash out without cause if they fail to meet our "standards." When this becomes a pattern, it will destroy relationships, and invariably block our blessings.

Anger not only predisposes us to physical disease, it is also an indicator that our mental health may be in jeopardy. For instance, depression can manifest itself as anger, particularly in men. In recent years, research has shown that the traditional tools used to screen for depression contain a strong bias toward women. This may explain why women are twice as likely as men to be diagnosed with depression. While depressed females are prone to manifest such typical symptoms as sadness and tearfulness, men with depression may not exhibit this kind of sadness. Instead they are more apt to display aggression, substance abuse, risk-taking behaviors, and anger. This further validates the strong connections between physical, emotional, and mental health.

Peace vs. stress

Stress is an unavoidable part of life. Thankfully, our bodies and minds are designed to handle it. In threatening situations the body releases various hormones and chemicals. These affect the cardiovascular system, the nervous system, the muscles—even the hair follicles! This intrinsic "fight or flight" body response equips us to either confront head-on whatever is causing the stress (i.e., "fight"), or run away! Our ability to deal with stress in this manner is not detrimental, but life preserving.

If this is the case, then what is so bad about stress? The problem lies in the nature and frequency of whatever is causing these hormones to be released. With prolonged stress, the same reaction that gives us strength and stamina to escape harm operates in situations that are in no way life threatening. Everyday stressors like stacks of unpaid bills or an overbearing boss are not the kinds of things we literally fight or run from (at least I hope not!). To make matters worse, day-to-day stress tends to be chronic. Under these conditions, the hormones and chemicals that help us respond to real threats get released into our bloodstreams constantly, even though we don't face threats. Such constant exposure is harmful rather than helpful.

There are many reasons why type 2 diabetes, obesity, depression, stroke, and heart disease become more common with age. And stress—particularly chronic, long-term stress—is included with all the other risk factors. For some people it plays a major role in the onset of these conditions, but other folks are not affected this way. The second category is comprised of people who (like everyone else) have lived through years of difficult times but successfully guarded themselves against the toxic effects of stress. They endure adversity without allowing it to take a toll on their bodies. Some would call them effective stress managers; I like to call them effective peace managers. In troubling times, they refuse to let circumstances govern them. Instead they allow a spirit of peace to "manage" their hearts. In this way, they preserve their overall health.

BIBLICAL INSIGHTS

And behold, there was a man in Jerusalem whose name was Simeon, and this man was just and devout, waiting for the Consolation of Israel, and the Holy Spirit was upon him. And it had been revealed to him by the Holy Spirit that he would not see death before he had seen the Lord's Christ. So he came by the Spirit into the temple, And when the parents brought in the Child Jesus, to do for Him according to the custom of the law, he took Him up in his arms and blessed God and said: "Lord, now You are letting Your servant depart in peace, according

to Your word; for my eyes have seen Your salvation
which You have prepared before the face of all
peoples, a light to bring revelation to the Gentiles,
and the glory of Your people Israel."
—LUKE 2:25–32

In my opinion, Simeon offers a supreme example of
stress management. The little we know about him
reveals other admirable traits, such as his devout and
patient character. Still, the brief passage of his life
recorded by Luke leaves the impression of someone
cool and collected. One attribute of people who deal
effectively with stress is their extreme selectiveness in
responding to stressors. Not many things disturb them,
or get them "off their square," so to speak. This helps
them stay calm, even in troubling times. The Bible
says Simeon had God's assurance that he would not
die before seeing the Messiah. Now how could *anything* make a person fret after receiving such a promise?
I imagine he confidently embraced his purpose and
worried little, if at all.

Further evidence of Simeon's calm demeanor comes
from him tuning in to the prompting of the Holy Spirit.
It's hard to hear God's voice when our minds are distracted, and stress is a major distraction. When the
time came for him to meet Jesus, Simeon heard the
voice of the Lord, who led him to the *right* place. When
we let stress prevail, we're bound to end up in the
wrong place! After his encounter with Christ, Simeon
declared the promise had been fulfilled and his mission accomplished. Simeon's story is simple. While not
full of fireworks, bells, and whistles, he fulfilled his
life's purpose and had peace in the end.

We become vulnerable to stress when we are not
confident of our purpose. However, many people feel
considerable confusion over the matter of "purpose."
Why is this so? Does God keep us in the dark? Does the
Holy Spirit want us pulled in different directions as we
blindly pursue our calling? Of course, the answer is no.

> The Bible says, "God is not the author of confusion but of peace..." (1 Cor. 14:33). Interestingly Paul wrote these words in the context of explaining church order and spiritual gifts. At the time, one cause for their confusion came from failing to understand their God-given purpose. The more things change, the more they stay the same! Sometimes we select our own life's purpose (with fireworks, bells, and whistles) and then credit it to God. We tune in to the desires of our flesh—or the prompting of other people—instead of the voice of the Holy Spirit. When we allow this to happen, we trade confidence for uncertainty, and tranquility for tension. Remember: following God's call always leads to peace; following our own "calling" will always lead to stress.

As mentioned earlier, the hormones and chemicals released in response to stress can have a damaging effect, especially when it is chronic. Here are a few ways, from a purely *physical* standpoint, to combat those effects:

- *Exercise regularly.* Stress clouds our thinking and makes us tense. A good workout combats both by helping release tension and clearing our minds so we keep things in a proper perspective. Exercise releases hormones that help us to relax and unwind. If done a few hours before bedtime, it improves the quality of sleep.

- *Get adequate sleep.* Stress will steal a good night's sleep. And when we are sleep deprived, the conditions causing the stress seem all the more intimidating. Sleep deprivation also makes us irritable, impairs our ability to make sensible decisions, and even increases our appetites.

- *Eat wisely.* Stress hormones are appetite stimulants. Unfortunately, when we feel overwhelmed, we tend to crave foods that are salty, sweet, and high in fat. "Stress eaters" typically reach for chips and cookies, not brown rice and kale. To make matters worse, when we are stressed, moderation falls by the wayside; we are likely to binge eat. In the end, we eat far too much of the wrong types of foods. The first step in combating this tendency is to recognize it. Watch what you eat and when! Plan trips to the supermarket, and be highly restrained once you get there. Make a list and stick to it. It's hard to indulge yourself with a whole container of ice cream if you've left it in the grocer's freezer!

These are great tips from a *physical* standpoint. Yet from a *spiritual* standpoint, the key to stress management begins with disciplining the mind. As with all attitudes and emotions, we have the capacity to *choose how we respond*. It is up to us to decide how life's circumstances will affect us. Either they will toss us to and fro like a boat in a stormy sea, or we will maintain our focus and refuse to give them the power to prevail. The choice is ours. Choose to be anchored.

BIBLICAL INSIGHTS

Oh, that my words were written! Oh, that they were inscribed in a book! That they were engraved on a rock with an iron pen and lead, forever! For I know that my Redeemer lives, and He shall stand at last on the earth; and after my skin is destroyed, this I know, that in my flesh I shall see God, whom I shall see for myself, and my eyes shall behold, and not another. How my heart yearns within me!
—Job 19:23–27

Stress is an unavoidable part of life. As long as we live, we will face stress in one form or another. Thankfully, we are able to handle most day-to-day challenges because they have one or more of the following characteristics:

- *They are modifiable.* When under extreme pressure or pulled in several directions, it is common to feel "locked in." Stress can consume us to the point of losing sight of our options. However, in reality most circumstances can be modified—at least to some extent. What are our options? There are several! For example, eliminate things from our "to do" list, downsize our lives, set boundaries on relationships, minimize outside commitments, find a new job, or learn to say no. While these can represent dramatic changes, they still illustrate my point: though we may feel bound by circumstances, quite often we are equipped to change them.

- *They can be lessened by moral support.* Friends, family, pastors, and health care providers are vital resources for help during stressful times. And nowadays most personnel departments even offer employees some form of assistance with stress management. Support systems may not *change* situations, but others' guidance and objective viewpoints can help us *resolve* them.

- *They carry a tinge of our own responsibility.* Stress often comes upon us because of poor choices. Unwise and hasty decisions (especially with respect to money) lead to unpleasant consequences. In some ways, knowing we are responsible is what sustains us. Stress, then, becomes a life coach, teaching us some valuable—albeit painful—lessons.

Each of these conditions helps keep us from becoming overwhelmed by stress. Yes, times may be difficult, but they need not consume us. Not so with Job. He didn't have any of the three options I just outlined. In the first two chapters of the book, we learn that a devastating succession of calamities struck him. This affected him emotionally, physically, and relationally—in ways that he was powerless to *modify*. We also learn the friends who should have offered him *support* instead made matters worse. Yet Job was in no way *responsible* for what happened to him. From his point of view, there was no logical explanation, yet he had the added stress of having to defend his innocence.

So what sustained Job? How did he get through such incomprehensible stress? He had eternal hope. At the height of despair, at the point he felt most overwhelmed, he uttered the words found in our verses. They beautifully affirmed his steadfast hope in God, our Redeemer. Although not perfect, Job's hope gave him the capacity to endure. Prayerfully, none of us will ever experience this kind of stress. However, through his example we gain insights on how to handle our personal trials. Never lose hope. Never forget our Redeemer yet lives!

Chapter 3

BONES AND MUSCLES

Strengthen the weak hands, and make firm the feeble knees.
—ISAIAH 35:3

"W ow, I can't believe you're ___ years old! You look great!" Who wouldn't like receiving such a compliment? Regardless of the number that fills in the blank—forty, sixty, eighty, or higher—we love to hear these kinds of words. Of course, there are many facets to aging gracefully, each of which can generate favorable comments. But one sure way to keep the flattery flowing is through preserving bones and muscles. Whatever you do, don't take them for granted.

In a passage from the Book of Job, Job cries out to God with a description of how he was created: "Did You not pour me out like milk, and curdle me like cheese, clothe me with skin and flesh, and knit me together with bones and sinews?" (Job 10:10–11). Job uttered these words at the height of his distress—mentally anguished, physically afflicted, and desperate for an explanation. His plea reminds me of a tendency in human nature: we are more likely to recognize how our "bones and sinews" are miraculously knit together when they *aren't* functioning properly. Still, we can take proactive measures early on that will help preserve them, which will enable us to experience the benefits as we grow older.

Stature, independence, and tackling stairs without intimidation are some of the advantages of having healthy bones and muscles. But it doesn't end there. In this chapter, let's first review a bit of basic physiology to understand their normal function. Then we'll discuss some of the changes commonly seen with aging—particularly changes in bones—and the best ways to combat them.

BONE

Paul uses the analogy of a building (more precisely, a temple) to describe the body:

> Or do you not know that your body is the temple of the Holy Spirit who is in you, whom you have from God, and you are not your own?
>
> —1 CORINTHIANS 6:19

He uses the same imagery to describe who we are as believers, bound to other followers of Christ like a building:

> Now, therefore, you are no longer strangers and foreigners, but fellow citizens with the saints and members of the household of God, having been built on the foundation of the apostles and prophets, Jesus Christ Himself being the chief cornerstone, in whom the whole building, being fitted together, grows into a holy temple in the Lord, in whom you also are being built together for a dwelling place of God in the Spirit.
>
> —EPHESIANS 2:19–22

If we compare ourselves to a building, then the skeleton is the framework. It determines height, the basic shape, and (most importantly) provides support for everything else. Unlike beams and girders, though, bone is living tissue. It is dynamic, not stagnant. As such, it has properties that would be coveted by any mechanical engineer:

- Stiff but flexible. Upright posture requires stiff bones; otherwise we would slump against gravity. However, our bodies are constantly subjected to all kinds of forceful impact. So a bone's stiffness must be balanced with the capacity to absorb energy without breaking. A healthy bone is able to shorten and widen when compressed, and lengthen and narrow when pulled. Brittle bones have stiffness but lack flexibility, which makes them prone to fracture.

- Lightweight but strong. If bones were dense and heavy, their added weight would restrict movement. Rather than possessing graceful agility, we would resemble Iron Man. Yet their lack of density doesn't compromise their strength. Bones support hundreds of pounds of flesh—all day, every day. Along with bearing our body weight, they sustain the forces generated through activities like pushing and lifting.

The unique composition and structure of bone gives it these properties. It contains both flexible tissue (collagen) and hard mineral (calcium), in varying proportions. The design is indeed an architectural masterpiece. The "blueprint" for the body's more than two hundred bones differs from one bone to the next. Some are dense and others are spongy, depending on location and function. And true to Job's description, some parts of bone marrow even look knitted.

As with other organs and tissues, the state of our bones is influenced by lifestyle—particularly nutrition, exercise, and avoiding tobacco. Our diets supply calcium and vitamin D, both essential components of healthy bones. Many foods contain calcium; dairy products are the richest source. Other calcium-rich foods include green leafy vegetables, nuts, beans, and molasses, especially for vegetarians. With vitamin D, diet is not the only source. Ergocalciferol, or vitamin D_2, is found in foods like oily fish. But cholecalciferol, or vitamin D_3, is produced by the skin in response to the sun's ultraviolet B rays. Inside the body, vitamin D behaves more like a hormone than a vitamin per se.

Of course, hormones affect a wide variety of tissues. So does vitamin D, with tissues throughout the body responding to it in some way. Ongoing research is shedding more light on the latter's role in such areas as cancer, autoimmune disorders, and cardiovascular disease. What medical experts do know is how vital vitamin D is to bone health. Because bone is dynamic, there is constant turnover and a constant need for a fresh supply of calcium. Vitamin D regulates the delivery of calcium from the intestines to the bloodstream and then to the bone. Without it we lose bone density and strength.

BIBLICAL INSIGHTS

I am dark, but lovely, O daughters of Jerusalem, like the tents of Kedar, like the curtains of Solomon. Do not look upon me, because I am dark, because the sun has tanned me. My mother's sons were angry with me; they made me the keeper of the vineyards, but my own vineyard I have not kept.

—SONG OF SOLOMON 1:5–6

The Shulamite maiden who spoke these words (and happened to be Solomon's first wife) would be a misfit among the women of today's culture. She would never stretch out at the poolside or along the beach, lowering her bathing suit straps to get an even tan. If she somehow could morph into this century, I can only imagine her amazement to find people *paying* to spend time in a tanning booth. She was not at all pleased—as seen by her anguish—about the sun's effect on her skin. She didn't choose to be exposed to those harsh rays, but had been victimized by a few angry brothers. We don't know the details of the conflict, but they punished this maiden by forcing her to work outside. Along with the tanning, she described her skin as being like the "tents of Kedar," which were fashioned from a coarse, weather-beaten fabric. The color and texture of her skin had changed.

Still, I bet her vitamin D levels were awesome! And herein lies a clinical dilemma—what I call the "metabolic-psychiatric-dermatologic" predicament (what a mouthful!). Clearly sun exposure offers health advantages, with vitamin D metabolism a great example of its benefits. Sun rays also contain mental health benefits. Many people with depression and other mood disorders are sensitive to lack of sunlight; winter months are difficult in part because of fewer daylight hours. Yet we must balance these benefits against the sun's harmful effects on the skin. While the Shulamite maiden's main issue was cosmetic, the increased risk of skin cancer due to excessive exposure is a more serious concern. In some people, especially those with fair skin, this risk offsets any benefit. Use good judgment, and consult your health care provider about this issue before heading outside. For people with a low cancer risk, a few minutes of bare skin exposure followed by sunscreen is generally OK. For those at high risk, sunscreen, long sleeves, and hats are in order. You can always take vitamin D (and even an antidepressant) in pill form.

The Institute of Medicine has made recommendations for how much calcium and vitamin D should be supplied through the diet during various stages of life. These levels help to preserve bone strength and prevent fractures:[1]

Population	Recommended Daily Dose	
	Vitamin D (IU)	Calcium (mg)
Women		
Aged 19–50	600	1,000
Aged 51–70	600	1,200
Aged > 70	800	1,200
Pregnant Women		
Aged < 18	600	1,300
Aged > 18	600	1,000
Breastfeeding women		
Aged < 18	600	1,300
Aged > 18	600	1,000

Population	Recommended Daily Dose	
	Vitamin D (IU)	Calcium (mg)
Men		
Aged 19–50	600	1,000
Aged 51–70	600	1,000
Aged > 70	800	1,200

Optimal bone health requires calcium and vitamin D. Both are supplied by the diet, along with exposure to sunlight for vitamin D. Calcium depends heavily on dairy products, which is not always practical because of lactose intolerance or food preferences. You can meet the latter via roughly fifteen minutes a day of unprotected skin exposure, several days per week. That means wearing a bathing suit, or shorts with a short sleeved shirt, *without* sunscreen. This of course is not possible in some areas (including the Midwest, where I live). And it must be balanced against the risks of skin damage and skin cancer.

Natural sources of nutrients are ideal. However, for a variety of reasons, people typically cannot obtain recommended intake of calcium and vitamin D from natural sources. This is why supplements are so common, especially among postmenopausal women. An estimated 60 percent of women over the age of sixty use supplements for vitamin D, calcium, or both. But many take daily doses far in excess of the recommended amount. They think that "more is better," and that high doses of supplements will ensure the bones stay strong with advancing age. While such reasoning makes a bit of sense in theory, the evidence says otherwise.

To address this issue, the US Preventive Services Task Force (USPSTF) reviewed data gleaned from large studies weighing the benefits, risks, and outcomes of calcium and vitamin D supplements. In 2013 they issued recommendations for fracture prevention based on these findings.[2] Keep in mind their recommendations apply to a specific group of people: men and women who live *in the community* (not in an assisted living facility, a nursing home, or other institutional setting), who do *not* have osteoporosis, who do *not* have vitamin D deficiency, and who have *not* had a bone fracture. If you fit those parameters, the Task Force recommends the following use of calcium and vitamin D supplements:

- Women *prior to* menopause, and men: There is *insufficient evidence* to support the use of supplements for preventing fractures.

- Women *after* menopause: There is *insufficient evidence* to support using supplements at a dose greater than 400 IU of vitamin D_3, and greater than 1,000 mg of calcium daily.

- Using supplements containing 400 IU or less of vitamin D_3 and 1,000 mg or less of calcium is *not recommended.*

With respect to men and younger women, the USPSTF did not find sufficient evidence either *for* or *against* the use of supplements for fracture prevention. The studies they analyzed did not show a net benefit in this particular group, which made it impossible to accurately assess the balance of potential benefits to potential harms. The same applied to postmenopausal women taking more than 400 IU of vitamin D3 and more than 1,000 mg of calcium. With the smaller doses, the data showed an increased risk of kidney stones, which is why the recommendation advises against their use.

Again, these recommendations apply to adults who live in the community and have healthy bones. The USPSTF does not deny the importance of calcium and vitamin D for bone health. But sound recommendations don't rely on intuition, assumption, or gut feelings—they must be backed by evidence. A final note worth mentioning is that in this particular set of guidelines, the issue of supplements for people with known dietary deficiencies is not addressed. I will address this topic later, specifically in instances where they have proven benefits.

BIBLICAL INSIGHTS

And He said to me, "Son of man, can these bones live?" So I answered, "O Lord GOD, You know."
—EZEKIEL 37:3

Ezekiel was a prophet to Israel during the time when its people were held captive in Babylon. God often reinforced His verbal communication to Ezekiel with vivid imagery and symbolism. One such instance appears in chapter 37, where the prophet travels in the spirit realm to a valley of dry bones. The gist of the message was hope to a nation displaced and fragmented, which had lost its way spiritually. On the surface they appeared as hopeless and forsaken as these dry bones. Yet all was not lost. God had the power to restore them and give them new life.

This is a beautiful word-picture, but on another level it reminds me of the importance of the *quality* of life, not just the *quantity*. Of course, we would all like to live for many years, but typically that desire correlates to retaining our strength and independence. Certainly, some degree of frailty is an inevitable part of aging. But don't allow yourself to become a "dry bone." In this passage the bones were not restored so they could lead aimless, ineffectual, tedious lives. God created them to serve as a great army full of power and purpose. Take measures to preserve your vitality on every front. Keep yourself spiritually, mentally, and physically alive!

MUSCLES

There are two basic types of muscle: smooth and skeletal. Smooth muscle is found on our internal organs—the type that makes our hearts beat and our stomachs churn. We don't *decide* whether or not we'll move our smooth muscles, nor do we need to set aside time to *work them out* as we do skeletal muscle. Our discussion, then, relates to skeletal muscle. In the analogy of a building or structure, we have to think of a mobile home. If bone represents the framework, then skeletal muscle would be the side panels and wheels. That's because skeletal muscle gives us form and allows us to move.

Muscle tissue comprises the largest organ of the body. Like bone, it is an architectural masterpiece. A muscle operates as a single unit (the biceps or the hamstring, for instance) but is made up of individual fibers. Each fiber, in turn, is comprised of smaller units called myofibrils. The myofibril responds to its own nerve and contains the proteins that do the actual work of contraction. All the components—proteins, nerves, myofibrils and fibers—are bound together in a neat package and attached to the bone via the tendon. The packaging is what gives the muscle its characteristic striated pattern.

If the *design* of muscle is an architectural masterpiece, then the *function* of muscle is a tour de force of physics and engineering. The fibers within a muscle are not all the same length and don't all run perfectly parallel to one another. Some are parallel; others are aligned at varying angles. Of course, design and function go hand in hand. The science of physics comes into play with respect to fiber length, alignment, and the way in which the muscle is attached to the bone or joint. If you're a physics buff, then you can appreciate such concepts as length-tension curves, contraction velocity, and the force-generating axis. All these work together to give us strength and the ability to move. Just thinking about it puts me in agreement with David, who said, "I will praise You, for I am fearfully and wonderfully made; marvelous are Your works, and that my soul knows very well" (Ps. 139:14).

Providing strength and mobility are not the muscles' only function. They also work to help regulate metabolism, which is especially important with respect to type 2 diabetes and prediabetes. These conditions are extremely common, with type 2 diabetes affecting about eighteen million adults in the United States, and prediabetes another eighty million. So what role do muscles play in offsetting this epidemic? They use glucose ("blood sugar") as their primary source of energy. Physical activity depletes their available stores of glucose, meaning they must replenish the supply. Insulin is the hormone responsible for getting glucose from the bloodstream into the muscles. Regular exercise brings about a heightened responsiveness to insulin, helping remove glucose from the bloodstream more efficiently. The hallmark for the early stages of type 2 diabetes and prediabetes is a state of "insulin resistance." This is what causes high levels of glucose in the bloodstream. So the "insulin sensitivity" produced by regular exercise is essential for controlling the blood sugar, even preventing type 2 diabetes and prediabetes.

BIBLICAL INSIGHTS

> Now Moses was tending the flock of Jethro his father-in-law, the priest of Midian. And he led the flock to the back of the desert, and came to Horeb, the mountain of God.
>
> —Exodus 3:1

The life span of Moses can be divided into three segments, each lasting forty years. He spent the first third in Egypt, where he was born. This particular verse reflects the second period, when Moses worked as a shepherd in Midian. Not an easy, sedentary job, we can assume that Moses walked, climbed, lifted, and even ran on a regular basis—over rugged terrain of rocks, hills, and mountains. A shepherd constantly searched for water and pasture. He ran after wandering sheep to carry them back to the fold. When threatened by wild animals, the shepherd defended the flock and chased predators away. In other words, exhausting, sweat-generating toil. Yet Moses didn't take on this occupation until the age of forty and kept at it until eighty.

One of the major effects of aging is that over time, muscle mass diminishes. This downward trend starts in the early forties. By eighty, people typically experience a 30 percent to 40 percent reduction in strength. However (and thankfully), muscle abides by the "use it or lose it" principle, meaning physical activity helps offset this decline. Yes, you should set aside time for regular exercise, but—as in the case of Moses—you can maintain strength through work-related and leisure time activities. Protein supplements will not change the size or strength of muscles, nor are they a substitute for a regular workout. When Moses turned eighty, the Lord presented him with a new "career opportunity." Even though it would require hard work and long hours on his feet, his regimen meant he could accept the position. Of course, Moses first told God that he wasn't the right man for the job. But his apprehension stemmed from fear and insecurity, not because of weakness or frailty. One of the primary reasons he was conditioned enough to lead the nation of Israel out of Egypt was because at forty—the age when muscle mass begins to decline—he kept himself fit!

Certainly time has an effect on all tissues of the body, bone and muscle included. Let's look at a couple of these changes and how to best prevent them, or at least delay their progression.

OSTEOPOROSIS

With osteoporosis, the bones become fragile due to a decline in their *quality* and *quantity*. The former relates to bone architecture and structure; the latter relates to bone density. Fragile bones are prone to break, which is why prevention and treatment are so vital. Hip fractures and fractures in the spine (vertebral fractures) are two of the most common sites for osteoporosis-related fractures. The *consequences* of fractures are significant. Along with pain, they commonly lead to long-term disability, loss of independence, and a significant decline in the quality of life.

While the fracture itself may not be life-threatening, sustaining a fracture increases the risk for other illnesses and death. About 25 percent of people who fracture their hips die within a year. An even larger percentage require extensive rehabilitation or must relocate to a nursing facility. Fractures pose an economic burden to an already strained health care system. By 2025 the projected annual cost of osteoporosis-related fractures is expected to exceed $25 billion.[3]

Given this forecast, measures to prevent and treat osteoporosis, and thereby reduce the incidence of fractures, are worthwhile on many fronts. The first step to prevention is recognizing risk factors. While some can be modified, others cannot. They include:

- Gender. Osteoporosis is more common in women than in men. About half of all women over age fifty will experience an osteoporosis-related fracture at some point in their lifetimes.

- Race. Osteoporosis is more likely to develop in people of Caucasian and Asian ancestry. This, however, should not give Hispanics and African Americans a false sense of security. Bone loss happens to people of every race.

- Age. In general, osteoporosis is a disease of older adults. When it develops in younger adults, secondary causes may play a role, some of which are listed in the next section.

- Genetics. Osteoporosis tends to run in families.

- Smoking. There is an established connection between tobacco use and bone loss. There is even some evidence that children exposed to secondhand smoke are more likely to develop osteoporosis in adulthood.

- Vitamin D deficiency.

- Low calcium intake.

- Alcohol abuse. This one is a two-edged sword. Alcohol increases the risk for osteoporosis through accelerating bone loss *and* it increases the risk for fractures, simply because people who drink tend to fall down more often than people who don't.

Several conditions (or their treatment) may lead to bone loss:

- Thyroid and parathyroid gland disease
- Frequent use of steroids
- Early menopause
- Amenorrhea (the absence of regular menstrual periods)
- Chronic lung disease
- Immobility
- Diabetes (types 1 and 2)
- Rheumatoid arthritis
- Systemic lupus erythematosus
- Ankylosing spondylitis
- Sex hormone deficiency
- Anorexia nervosa
- Adrenal gland disease
- Inflammatory bowel disease
- Celiac disease
- Gastric bypass surgery

Prevention

If proverbs were assigned to diseases, then "An ounce of prevention is worth a pound of cure" would get tagged to osteoporosis. When it comes to bone health, good habits started early in life pay great dividends in the long run. Bone is not a stagnant tissue. Throughout life, there is constant turnover with construction coupled to destruction. This attribute of bone makes for good news and bad news. The good news is that it's never too late to start practicing good habits, because bones are in a perpetual state of formation. The bad news is that over time, the rate of growth—compared to the rate of destruction—changes. In our younger years, there is a lot more building; in older years, there is more tearing down. So while a healthy lifestyle at *any* age is great for the bones, the maximum benefit is achieved when you implement healthy habits in childhood.

So what can we do—and encourage our children and grandchildren to do—to help preserve bone strength? As is the case with heart disease and cancer prevention, three areas are key: diet, physical activity, and breaking bad habits.

- Diet: Calcium and vitamin D are essential for healthy bones. Along with dairy products, other sources include green leafy vegetables (e.g., broccoli, kale, brussels sprouts), nuts, beans, and fish with edible bones (e.g., sardines, salmon). For many people, dietary sources are insufficient because of food preferences or lactose intolerance. Likewise, exposure to sunlight as a source of vitamin D is sometimes not feasible. In such instances, supplements can be used to fill in the gaps.

  Over-the-counter calcium supplements come in several formulations. Calcium carbonate and calcium citrate are more common than calcium lactate and calcium gluconate. The labels usually include total milligrams and elemental milligrams. The elemental calcium is used to determine daily requirements.

  Calcium carbonate has a relatively high elemental calcium content but is more likely to cause bloating and constipation than other preparations. You should take it with meals, because stomach acid improves the absorption. Calcium citrate provides less elemental calcium, but it has fewer side effects and can be taken with or without food.

Remember calcium supplements should be used to make up the difference when dietary sources are not enough. If the composition of the diet meets the recommended daily allowance, then there is no need to take supplements. If the diet is inadequate, then the dose of the supplement should only make up the difference—not exceed the recommendation. If you need more than five hundred milligrams, split the dosing into twice a day. This helps optimize absorption.

There is no specific test to check whether or not the calcium intake is adequate. Doctors are limited to assessing the diet. Yes, calcium levels can be checked in the bloodstream, but this measurement does not help in determining whether the diet is sufficient or if supplements are needed. However, this is not the case with vitamin D, where a simple blood test can screen for deficiencies. If the vitamin D blood level is low, your health care provider will decide whether you need a prescription-strength supplement or if an over-the-counter formula will suffice. Many calcium supplements now include vitamin D.

- Physical activity. Regular exercise, particularly the weight-bearing kind, helps to preserve bone density. When the muscle contracts, it pulls against the bone and stimulates its growth. Keep in mind that while exercise is beneficial, overtraining can be detrimental. When the workout regimen is so rigorous that a woman or girl misses her menstrual period, then the risk for osteoporosis *increases* rather than *decreases*.

- Bad habits. Smoking and excessive alcohol consumption both contribute to osteoporosis. With smoking the connection is clear, yet assessing the independent contribution of tobacco is a bit complicated. This is because other variables cloud the picture.

Consider that people who smoke tend to be thin and less physically active, often because of the lung and heart problems caused by smoking. Women who smoke are likely to experience early menopause. People who smoke often have dietary deficiencies, including calcium. And people who smoke also drink more than people who don't. Each one of these factors poses an independent risk for osteoporosis. So while the *risk* from smoking is indisputable, the *magnitude* of the risk can be difficult to determine. The bottom line is this—if you want healthy bones, don't smoke!

Meanwhile, excessive alcohol consumption disrupts the fine-tuned system that keeps calcium in balance. Alcohol has a negative impact on various hormones that work to regulate calcium and the production of vitamin D. People who are "under the influence" are prone to fall and injure themselves. As Proverbs says: "Who has wounds without cause? Who has redness of eyes? Those who linger long at the wine" (Prov. 23:29–30). And of the many types of osteoporosis-related fractures, people who drink are more likely to sustain hip fractures—the most serious kind.

BIBLICAL INSIGHTS

She girds herself with strength, and strengthens her arms.

—Proverbs 31:17

The last chapter of the Book of Proverbs describes a phenomenal woman, one we affectionately call "The

Virtuous Woman." This girl has it all! She's a great mom, a superb wife, and a thoughtful boss to her servants. She is diligent, conscientious, kind, wise, resourceful, efficient—the list of positive attributes goes on and on. It's enough to give us regular women an inferiority complex! And to top it off, she's in great shape. According to verse 17, her arms are strong. I can imagine even in her middle-age and senior years there was noticeable definition in her biceps, triceps, and deltoid muscles. If she were to dress in modern fashions, she would face no shame in going sleeveless. Isn't it interesting that in a chapter devoted to her excellent character, the Holy Spirit found it necessary to mention she was physically fit? What a confirmation to the truth that God is interested in our total being—body, mind, and spirit.

Diagnosis, screening, and treatment

Low bone mineral density defines both osteoporosis and osteopenia. In the latter condition, bone density is less than normal, but not quite to the extent of osteoporosis. Bone density is measured using the dual-energy x-ray absorptiometry (DEXA) scan. The results from the scan help generate a number known as a "T-score" (for postmenopausal women and men older than fifty) or a "Z-score" (for premenopausal women and younger men). The T-score is determined by analyzing the individual's bone mineral density in comparison to that of a thirty-year-old. As density diminishes, the score becomes more and more negative. The cutoffs for osteopenic and osteoporotic bones are set at the standard deviations from the norm. They are defined by the following criteria:

- A T-score minus 2.5 or lower is osteoporosis

- A T-score between minus 1.0 and minus 2.5 is osteopenia

- A T-score of minus 1.0 or higher is normal

Women over age sixty-five should be screened with a DEXA scan. Younger women and men are also candidates for screening, depending on their age and other risk factors. Talk to your health care provider to determine if screening is right for you.

Regardless of the T-score or the DEXA scan results, a physician also makes an osteoporosis diagnosis when an individual suffers a hip or vertebral fracture. When someone sustains a fracture in other areas—for instance, the wrist or forearm—then the diagnosis rests on clinical judgment. If a bone other than the hip or spine breaks, and the force causing the break was minimal or would not have typically broken a "normal" bone, then the criteria for osteoporosis is met again, albeit subjectively. These are known as "fragility fractures."

With most medical conditions, a doctor defers treatment until the diagnosis is sealed by some sort of objective test or through clinical judgment. And this applies to osteoporosis. But in recent years there has been a move toward assessing a person's *overall risk for fractures* to determine whether to start medications. This approach incorporates clinical information into the decision, and not just the T-score. Factors such as alcohol use, family history, steroid use, body weight, and smoking are taken into account to generate a score which estimates the likelihood that a person will break a bone over a ten-year period. If the score is high, treatment should be considered, even if the T-score is not that bad. One such tool is the Fracture Risk Assessment (FRAX), released in 2008 by the World Health Organization and available online at http://www.shef.ac.uk/FRAX/.

Treatment for osteoporosis starts with minimizing risk factors, and ensuring sufficient calcium and vitamin D intake. Medications are not a substitute for these fundamental measures. Currently there are several *choices* for medications but not too many *categories* of medications. Most of them work in the same way. However, research in this area is ongoing. Over the next few years, we can expect pharmaceutical companies to develop more therapies to broaden our options. Presently, the following drugs are approved:

MEDICATION (trade name)	ROUTE	DOSE
BISPHOSPHONATES		
Alendronate (Fosamax)	Oral	10 mg daily or 70 mg weekly
Risedronate (Actonel)	Oral	5 mg daily or 35 mg weekly
Zoledronic acid (Reclast)	Intravenous	5 mg yearly
Ibandronate (Boniva)	Oral	150 mg monthly
	Intravenous	3 mg every 3 months
OTHER AGENTS		
Raloxifene (Evista)	Oral	60 mg daily
Calcitonin (Miacalcin, Fortical)	Nasal	200 IU daily
	Subcutaneous	100 IU daily or every other day
Denosumab (Prolia)	Subcutaneous	60 mg every 6 months
Teriparatide (Forteo)	Subcutaneous	20 mg daily

The majority of medications for osteoporosis are antiresorptive, meaning they slow down the process whereby bones are resorbed. The bisphosphonates are in this category. Remember, bone is active tissue in a constant state of construction and destruction. The antiresorptive drugs work by inhibiting a specific type of cell known as the osteoclast. These are the cells responsible for breaking down or dissolving the bone. Oral and intravenous forms are available and are approved for both the treatment and prevention of osteoporosis. The most common side effects of the bisphosphonates are stomach upset and heartburn with oral use, and fever and flu-like symptoms with intravenous dosing.

Several other medications are available that have different forms of action. Raloxifene affects the tissues' estrogen receptors. The hormone calcitonin is involved in bone metabolism and calcium regulation. Denosumab affects the development and survival of osteoclasts. Teriparatide works by increasing bone mass. Each form of treatment carries its own risks, benefits, and side effects, so the choice of therapy must be tailored to the individual. Questions remain regarding how long a person should continue therapy and how often the bone density should be reassessed with a DEXA scan.

Muscle Atrophy

With osteoporosis comes a loss of bone strength. Muscle loses its strength and power through the process of atrophy. Both are manifestations of aging. Some degree of prevention is possible with both, and both carry significant risks if left unchecked. When muscle mass declines, it causes a concomitant loss of strength and a reduction in the muscle's capacity to use oxygen. Muscle loss beyond a critical threshold is called *sarcopenia*. This is the point where the likelihood of functional impairment and disability skyrockets.

Muscle mass is best preserved with adequate nutrition and physical activity. The latter entails structured exercise and an active lifestyle. As I said earlier, muscles follow the "use it or lose it" rule. People who follow a lifelong pattern of regular physical activity tend to live longer, mainly because of exercise's beneficial effects on chronic disease. Interestingly, several research studies have confirmed that it is never too late to reap the rewards. Men and women who don't start any exercise program until they are middle-aged still experience benefits. Our bodies were *made to move*. Not only is a sedentary lifestyle damaging to overall health; it is certainly not good for the muscles.

Physical activity is a key element to aging gracefully. We will revisit the topic of exercise in subsequent chapters. For now, let's discuss the problems of frailty and falls, which are potentially life-threatening consequences of muscle atrophy and sarcopenia.

FRAILTY

In our common vernacular, *frailty* refers to weakness and infirmity. But frailty, as described by Linda P. Fried and colleagues, is also a specific clinical syndrome occurring in some older adults.[4] Frailty increases the likelihood of disability, loss of independence, hospitalization, poor health outcomes, and even death. This syndrome is defined by specific criteria. Three of the following five meet the definition of frailty; two of the five constitute pre-frailty:

- Low grip strength
- Slowed walking speed
- Low physical activity
- Low energy
- Unintentional weight loss

Weakness is the most common initial manifestation of frailty. Low energy and weight loss typically follow weakness and rarely occur in its absence. Unlike with chronic *medical* conditions, where we know unequivocally that physical activity is beneficial, the data is not as solid with respect to the frailty syndrome. Although studies confirm that exercise definitely improves muscle strength, range of motion, and mobility, there is less convincing evidence that these improvements will suffice in preventing frailty. This speaks to its complexity, and the many variables outside of muscle mass that play a role in disability. As with other areas in aging, research is ongoing. In the meantime it would be erroneous to conclude that exercise is unimportant. Remember sedentary living is hazardous to our health.

FALLS

Falls are the leading cause of injury in seniors. About 40 percent of adults over sixty-five who reside in the community fall at least once a year; the numbers are higher for nursing home residents. Thankfully, most falls cause only minor injuries. But a significant number of people who fall (about 5 percent to 10 percent) sustain cuts, fractures, and head trauma.

Strong muscles help to keep us *off* the floor, and allow us to get up *from* the floor should we find ourselves there. Of course, some risk factors for falling have nothing to do with muscle strength. Such things as throw rugs, slippery shoes, inadequate lighting, poor vision, and medications with a sedative effect can all play a role. Even frisky pets might cause us to lose our footing. But clearly, muscle weakness is a major component. And weak muscles not only increase the odds of falling, they also increase the likelihood of sustaining a fracture.

So who is at risk for falling down? Certainly anyone who has ever fallen has a high chance of falling again. Any condition that impairs gait and mobility will increase the likelihood. Arthritis, neurological disorders and even obesity can affect balance and predispose to falls. The timed "Get-Up-and-Go" test is a useful tool for assessing the risk.[5] This simple test measures the time it takes a person to rise from an armchair, walk ten feet, turn around, walk back to the chair, and sit down. Most healthy adults over sixty years old can do this in less than ten seconds. However, it takes longer when a person has problems with gait, balance, strength, and mobility—all of which contribute to falls.

Exercise is useful for preventing falls, and some medical groups recommend vitamin D supplements. The exercise routine should include aerobic activities, along with strength training. Certainly the function of vitamin D in calcium metabolism and bone health is established, but vitamin D also plays a role in maintaining muscle mass. People with deficiencies are more prone to weakness, balance problems, and falls. As with all sorts of nutrients, it may not follow that taking a supplement will reduce the problem. At this writing, the USPSTF and the American Geriatrics Society recommend vitamin D supplements (800–1000 IU daily) for older adults who have ever fallen or who are at risk for falling. However, a large analysis of the available research was conducted after the introduction of these recommendations, and the findings did not show any benefit. People taking supplements fell down with the same frequency as those who didn't use them.

While the vitamin D question may be open for debate, there is no argument about the advantages of exercise. They are tremendous! The risks of disease, disability, injuries, and even death are lower in people who exercise regularly. It is beneficial to our physical as well as our mental health. Despite these advantages, the vast majority of adults do not meet the recommended amount of physical activity. For years I have treated men and women of all ages with problems like heart disease, type 2 diabetes, hypertension, and osteoarthritis. All of these (and many more) are potentially preventable. Even if not prevented, lifestyle modification will help better control them.

The "bottom line" here is that when we embrace sedentary living, we essentially *prevent* the chance for *prevention!* We close the door on strength and vitality, and open the door to disease and disability. Lack of exercise promotes a vicious circle, starting with weight gain that causes pain in the knees, which hinders activity, and the decline in activity leads to weight gain. And the same circle is true with many other conditions. But guess what? We can break that cycle! The first step, no matter what our age, is to get up and move! Once you get up, look for opportunities to use your muscles—even those as mundane as walking up a flight of stairs.

BIBLICAL INSIGHTS

Now behold, two of them were traveling that same day to a village called Emmaus, which was seven miles from Jerusalem.

—LUKE 24:13

Before the age of the push-button, labor-saving devices, drive-everywhere lifestyle, day-to-day living provided people with plenty of exercise. Health clubs and fitness centers didn't become popular until the second half of the twentieth century. Prior to that, the average person stayed physically active by default. In this passage Luke describes an incident that occurred after the death and resurrection of Jesus Christ. These travelers encounter Christ, who joins them in their journey, and even spends time in fellowship with them. As a detail-driven physician, Luke paints a clear picture. He gives such specifics as the number of men travelling, the name of the village they were headed for, and one more interesting point— the length of their journey.

I find this fascinating. Barring a hiking trip or a walking marathon, I can't remember ever setting out on foot for a destination seven miles away. Along with most Americans, I would jump in a car, a taxi, or a bus, even for half the distance! Surely times have changed. Industry and technology have given us conveniences our forefathers couldn't imagine. But there are pros and cons to this. The downside of modernism is the development of our sedentary culture. The average person spends about nineteen hours each day in either a chair or the bed. This level of inactivity has wreaked havoc on our health. It has ushered in (or exacerbated) modern afflictions—heart disease, type 2 diabetes, obesity, arthritis, and depression, to name a few. Our health is too valuable to jeopardize! Take advantage of every opportunity to stay on your feet. A nice, long walk is not only good for your health, but (at least for the men headed to Emmaus) it can be a great time to fellowship with the Lord!

Chapter 4

COMMUNITY AND SOCIAL NETWORKS

So continuing daily with one accord in the temple,
and breaking bread from house to house, they ate
their food with gladness and simplicity of heart.

—ACTS 2:46

M Y OLDEST SISTER lived in California for just over a decade. She and her husband bought a house in a sprawling development just outside of Los Angeles, built during the real estate boom of the late 1990s. I can still remember our mother's reaction. She absolutely loved the house—especially the bedroom and bath set aside for her. My sister extended an open invitation, an ideal setup for Mom to avoid Chicago's harsh winters. However, Mom had a problem with the layout of the "neighborhood," starting with the spacious distances between the houses. Nor did she care for the three-sided brick walls surrounding each one. We grew up in a neighborhood of unattached garages and chain-link fences. Mom complained these brick "fences" obscured the view of the "neighbors'" homes—which were too far away in the first place!

I laughed over retellings of the ensuing conversations when Mom, part of the Greatest Generation, attempted to explain "what's wrong with this picture" to my sister, a prototypical Baby Boomer. They were the original Point and Counterpoint!

- "You can't see your neighbors?" — "I don't need to see my neighbors."

- "Their kids won't be able to play in your yard." — "I don't want their kids playing in my yard."

- "What if you need something like a couple of eggs or a cup of sugar?" — "That's why we have grocery stores, Mom."

Over the years our nation's concepts of neighborhood have changed. Yet regardless of our birth generation, we cannot underestimate the benefits of strong, stable communities. In the not too distant past, the term *village* became a buzzword, signifying an environment with deep roots and wholesome relationships. The village is where a collective body of people, most of whom are not blood relatives, help to nurture one another and establish identity.

When we consider the value of strong communities, we are prone to focus on children—the advantages of good schools, safe parks, and the like for youngsters. But it turns out the rewards extend beyond childhood. Whether young or old, every age group reaps the benefits. Yes, children benefit from a good education and safe recreational opportunities. But for older folks, a strong social network—meaning flesh-and-blood connections, not electronic "friends" and "likes"—improves health and promotes longevity.

Recent research confirms this. For seniors, extreme loneliness increases the risk of death by nearly 15 percent. It brings about a decline in mental and physical health, with an impact on the latter estimated to be twice as high as that of obesity. It also generates stress. The chronic release of stress hormones (like cortisol) ushers in a myriad of health problems. Among the consequences of loneliness are elevated blood pressure, disrupted sleep, depression, and even alterations in the immune system.

Now, *loneliness* is not the same as *being alone*. In and of itself, physical isolation does not adversely affect health. In other words, it's OK to live alone, but it's not OK to be lonely. (One obvious exception is for those prone to falls and injuries, since people who live by themselves don't have access to immediate assistance.) It is not *physical* isolation but the sense of *social* isolation that impacts health. Unfortunately, some of the changes that come with age make matters worse. Impaired hearing, poor vision, decreased mobility, and losing the capacity to drive all have a "disconnecting" effect.

Still, there is good news. While loneliness is detrimental, positive social ties are protective to physical and mental well-being. Socially engaged seniors are more resilient, since satisfying relationships enhance our ability to bounce back from adversity. So the "village" concept turns out to be a necessary component of aging gracefully. In this chapter we'll first cover two aspects of community—work and worship—and then close with the topic of social networks.

BIBLICAL INSIGHTS

> On the third day there was a wedding in Cana of Galilee, and the mother of Jesus was there. Now both Jesus and His disciples were invited to the wedding. And when they ran out of wine, the mother of Jesus said to Him, "They have no wine."
> —JOHN 2:1–3

In his Gospel, John records eight miracles that confirm the deity of Christ. These verses give the setting of the first miracle: Jesus turning water into wine at a wedding feast. John doesn't relate whether the bride was a relative or if the groom's family extended the invitation. They may have just been friends. However, while there's much we *don't* know about this wedding, there's quite a bit we *do* know. It's clear the couple invited lots of people, including Jesus, His mother, and His disciples. The healthy quantity of wine consumed indicates the crowd's ample size. Jesus made enough to fill six water pots, each with a capacity of twenty to thirty gallons, *after* the guests drank the original batch! In this era, a wedding feast could last several days. It was a *community* event where the village celebrated together and shared the couple's joy. This ancient culture included expectations of a gracious, generous host. Running out of *anything* would have been a catastrophe! So Jesus's contribution was vital, since His miracle prevented a social disaster and made the occasion one to remember for eternity.

All four Gospel writers describe miracles that Christ performed. Certainly, these wonders impacted the lives of countless individuals. He healed the sick, restored sight to the blind, and cleansed lepers. Yet isn't it interesting that the first miracle John records did not help an individual per se, but occurred for the sake of the community? Relationships are important to God. Never underestimate the value of social ties, which are vital to our health and an essential component of graceful aging.

WORK

Work sets the foundation for thriving communities. High unemployment contributes to poverty, despair, and increased crime. As the socioeconomic status of a community declines, so does its health, increasing the rate of premature death by as much as 20 percent. This is why a person's zip code is a reliable predictor of his or her health status. Impoverished areas have higher rates of just about every affliction—heart disease, obesity, type 2 diabetes, cancer, mental illness, and infant mortality, to name a few.

Conversely, communities thrive on high employment rates. Not only does work produce tax revenue for a municipality, but their earnings potential instills a sense of satisfaction in its residents. Meaningful goals replace restlessness and discontentment. Health indicators improve, crime subsides, and despair lifts. It is no surprise that the wise King Solomon said "money answers everything" (Eccles. 10:19). We could go on with an extended discussion relating employment to health, sociology, and even politics. Instead, let's review two particular aspects: relationships and retirement.

Some of our strongest ties are formed in the workplace, especially a generation or two ago, when people didn't change jobs as frequently. According to *Forbes*, today's average worker remains at the same job for a little over four years. In surveys, 90 percent of the Millennial Generation (those born between the early 1980s and early 2000s) say they expect to stay with the same employer for less than three years. It's not entirely clear why people change jobs (and even careers) so frequently. Maybe because employer pension plans were more common several years ago. Unlike today's 401(k)s that will "roll over" from place to place, pension plans provided a strong incentive to stay put.

An advantage to keeping one job over the long term is how it fosters the creation of deep relationships in the workplace. Televisions shows from past generations reflect this: Laverne DeFazio and Shirley Feeney, Andy Griffith and Barney Fife, and even the crew of the USS Enterprise had ties that extended beyond their "9 to 5." These kinds of relationships provide an incalculable benefit—work generates more than a mere paycheck. One senior I spoke with offered an eloquent description of his coworkers: "These are the people I 'do life' with." I think he sized it up well.

BIBLICAL INSIGHTS

And as He walked by the Sea of Galilee, He saw Simon and Andrew his brother casting a net into the sea; for they were fishermen. Then Jesus said to them, "Follow Me, and I will make you become fishers of men." They immediately left their nets and followed Him. When He had gone a little farther from there, He saw James the son of Zebedee, and John his brother, who also were in the boat mending their nets. And immediately He called them, and they left their father Zebedee in the boat with the hired servants, and went after Him.

—Mark 1:16–20

Jesus called twelve men from a variety of occupations to shift gears and take on a new profession. The four in this passage happened to be fishermen. I imagine if Jesus had an HR department, His recruiter would trademark the slogan "Fishers of Men" and use it to brand the company. The twelve disciples formed relationships for life. They shared experiences that ran the gamut: they were together for Peter's mother-in-law's illness, dealt with conflict within the ranks, shared countless meals together, and even had to deal with Judas's heinous betrayal. Of course, they had a great "Supervisor" who created a work environment conducive to meaningful, lasting relationships. While they had the earthly "job" of disciples, they formed supernatural bonds that sealed them together until the end. What a great example of the blessings that come from workplace relationships.

A new concept

So if being employed offers so many benefits—supporting communities, creating resources, and strengthening relationships—then why would anyone choose to retire? Of course I'm being facetious, but only to a certain extent! (Before we go any further, let me clarify that being a homemaker and/or a stay-at-home parent constitutes work. You just don't fill out as many forms your first day!)

Throughout history, people have adjusted their activities as they grew older so their duties matched their capacities. Yet their duties didn't vanish at a predetermined age. Besides, the concept of "retirement" is fairly new, having originated during the twentieth century. President Franklin Roosevelt signed the Social Security Board (later the Social Security Administration) into federal law in 1935. So it is likely some readers of this book were born when Social Security as we know it didn't exist. Even age sixty-five happened to be chosen rather arbitrarily. It stemmed from two factors. First, a fair number of existing pension plans (private and public) used either sixty-five or seventy to gauge retirement age. Secondly, when the Committee on Economic Security looked at actuarial data, sixty-five worked best with respect to taxation and sustainability. (The Social Security Administration has a fascinating website on its history at www.ssa.gov/history.)

In addition, there is no *biblical* precedent for retirement. Being productive adds value to our days, while making a contribution—however small—is vital to our sense of identity. So it is no surprise that research shows retirement may be detrimental to your health! One study several years ago followed more than one thousand employees of Shell Oil Company after they retired. The investigators found the men and women who took an "early retirement" at age fifty-five doubled their risk of death before they reached sixty-five, compared to those who worked beyond age sixty.[1] Surely with advancing age and capacity we are permitted to slow down, but God forbid we stop.

BIBLICAL INSIGHTS

In the six hundredth year of Noah's life, in the second month, the seventeenth day of the month, on that day all the fountains of the great deep were broken up, and the windows of heaven were opened. And the rain was on the earth forty days and forty nights.
—GENESIS 7:11–12

I know dozens of people who are literally counting the days until retirement. Some are nearing sixty-five, but others are taking advantage of "early retirement" options offered by their employers. Invariably I'll ask such people two questions:

- "What do you plan on doing?"
- "Why are you retiring?"

The first question is important because retirees can easily slip into "couch potato" mode. If your job entails being on your feet and moving most of the day, you need to replace that activity. Otherwise, everything will start creeping higher: blood pressure, blood sugar, and especially body weight. Even aches and pains will escalate from sitting around all day.

The second question speaks to motive. Whether age fifty-five or sixty-five, people choose to retire for a number of reasons. While some are valid, others are dubious at best! Just for fun, consider how Noah's life lines up with some of the more common explanations:

- "I'm too old for this job." Really? Compared to whom? Noah stayed on the job in his sixth century, and worked it with gusto!

- "This job is too stressful." I would be the first to acknowledge that too much stress is bad for your health. But everything is relative. What one person calls stressful, another would call a piece of cake. Without question, Noah operated in a high-stress environment! Can you imagine being surrounded by *really wicked* people—all day, every day? By the grace of God he handled it and didn't quit.

- "My boss keeps changing my job description." Sometimes, especially when companies downsize, you get handed duties you never expected. Many people don't appreciate an expanded job description, so they retire. Consider, though, how Noah's kept growing. His "Boss" needed him to be a preacher, lumberjack, draftsman, carpenter, insulation specialist, zookeeper, weatherman, mariner, ornithologist, cattleman, farmer, and vintner. He did it all without complaining.

So if you feel frustrated at work and think about quitting, remember Noah. His faith—and phenomenal work ethic—are worth emulating. And whether you choose to retire or keep punching in, remember "whatever you do, do it heartily, as to the Lord and not to men, knowing that from the Lord you will receive the reward of the inheritance; for you serve the Lord Christ" (Col. 3:23–24).

WORSHIP

Religion serves as a hub for communities. In America, because we are blessed with religious freedom, diverse faiths form a "community mosaic," especially in large urban areas. When I worked in the central part of Chicago, my drive to the office took me through Jewish, Catholic, and Muslim neighborhoods—pockets of people bound by a common belief. I'm sure some vibrant communities contain a healthy sprinkling of atheists, but we cannot overlook how religion plays an important role in neighborhood vitality.

Religion contributes to health and longevity as well. Several medical studies verify the link between religion and health. It is a complex area to investigate because so many other factors may help explain the connection. For example, religious people might live longer because they are less likely to smoke and drink. Yet even when researchers tease out the variables, the benefits remain. Study after study confirms them, such as data from the Women's Health Initiative, which I first mentioned in chapter 2. It showed that women ages fifty and older who attended religious services every week were 20 percent less likely to die in any given year, compared to those who never attended. The advantage appeared even among those who occasionally skipped services. Women who averaged less frequent attendance still had a 15 percent lower death rate. There is also evidence that what we do once we get to church influences health. One study showed that seniors who routinely provided emotional support to other church members had a lower risk of death than those on the receiving end.

Religious commitment varies depending on age. In the typical Christian church, even though a range of ages is represented, seniors typically top the list when it comes to regular attendance. A 2010 Gallup poll assessing the number of people attending church by age found the following results:

- Age sixty-five and older: 53 percent.

- Age fifty to sixty-four: 43 percent.

- Age thirty to forty-nine: 41 percent.

- Age eighteen to twenty-nine: 35 percent.[2]

Certainly some congregations appeal to younger people. However, the church generally parallels the population—both are aging. And for many churches this is a source of great concern.

Now in her midseventies, my cousin has been a member of the same church her entire life. She was baptized there, married there, and one day expects her funeral will be held there. She and her husband have deep roots in the congregation and are actively involved in leadership.

Once she approached my husband for advice about a "serious" problem facing their congregation. She looked so solemn he thought my cousin's pastor had possibly mismanaged church funds or been involved in an extramarital affair. But this had nothing to do with any pastoral breech of integrity. She and other leaders were seriously concerned about the congregation's sustainability. With the average age of half their members over fifty, lately they'd had more funerals than births and marriages combined.

My husband first reassured her this situation was not unique to their congregation. For better or worse, over the years the concept of "church" has changed dramatically. At the time my cousin was born, a strong sense of allegiance existed among the members of most congregations—something I would describe as an "ownership interest." Now a new dynamic has surfaced where people attend "this" church or "that" church but are less likely to regard it as "my" church. Some even tie their membership solely to the current pastor: "I go to Rev. So-and-So's church."

The end result is that transient membership is the new norm. Millennials, who expect to experience several changes of jobs—even careers—switch churches almost as often as they do jobs. This explains why marketing and promotion have become such a huge factor in church sustainability, to the extent that advertising is included in the annual budgets of many congregations. This philosophy of promoting church is a fairly new concept. When my cousin was born, advertising was for salesmen, not pastors!

SENIOR SHORTCOMINGS

My husband acted wisely in not taking my cousin's congregation completely off the hook. Yes, transient members are a problem, but *not the only one*. When it comes to maintaining membership, each age group presents its own set of challenges to the congregation as a whole, including seniors. Unfortunately if *we* aren't aging gracefully, then neither will our churches. Here are five areas where Boomers and older folks are prone to miss the mark:

1. Respecting leadership

This is particularly a problem when the pastor is young or new to the pulpit. Be careful to avoid showing any signs of disrespect. Even a person's body language—especially during a sermon—speaks volumes. One of the first things a visitor observes is how the congregation treats the pastor. This can determine whether they join or keep on looking.

In his first letter to Timothy, Paul wrote, "Let no one *despise* your youth, but be an example to the believers in word, in conduct, in love, in spirit, in faith, in purity" (1 Tim. 4:12, emphasis added). Paul placed Timothy in a position of leadership at the church in Ephesus. However, he faced a problem. Not from lack of preparation; Paul had mentored him and ensured Timothy had adequate training and equipping. The problem stemmed from his relative youth. Only in his thirties, Pastor Timothy had stepped into a culture that equated age with wisdom. Apparently the seniors had a problem with that, reflected by Paul's use of *despise*. This is pretty strong language, which speaks to the level of disrespect Timothy endured. And Paul's words weren't just for Timothy. The problem of disrespect, especially coming from seniors, is universal nearly two thousand years later.

Like Timothy, my husband became a pastor in his thirties. Some of his greatest obstacles arose from elderly folks who just refused to listen to anyone younger. Thank God that during those early years, the majority of seniors were wonderfully supportive and absolute angels! Yet it took only a few "despisers" to plant seeds of discouragement. Oddly enough, I don't think they even realized the disrespect they projected. So, it is time for a self-assessment. Ask yourself, "Do I treat any young leaders in my congregation with deference? Or do I despise them?"

2. Being closed minded

Sometimes church growth and sustainability requires a modification in format, whether worship music, visitation programs, or various procedures. Things done in decades past may need to be revised and updated. Since we find comfort in the familiar, seniors often pose the greatest barrier to change. Remember, the *message* of the gospel is never revised. But anything else is fair game for change.

3. Welcoming new people

My husband and I used to joke about a common attitude of older church members, especially those in smaller congregations. While all *professed* a desire for growth, their actions revealed an *us four and no more* mentality. New people were barely recognized. While longtime members got a hug and warm conversation, newer folks were lucky to get a handshake and a cold "hello." And when they didn't come back, nobody noticed. Ironically the goal to increase membership rolls always stayed at the top of such churches' strategic plans.

4. Recognizing shortcomings

We strive to get *better* with age, but we don't become *perfect*! Sometimes seniors act as though they are exempt from church discipline. Irrespective of age, however, we all stand in need of a reprimand now and then. Don't take offense; age does not preclude correction.

A prime biblical example comes from Acts: "Then Ananias, hearing these words, fell down and breathed his last. So great fear came upon all those who heard these things" (Acts 5:5). Soon after the birth of the church came the need to confront error and carry out church discipline. (The more things change, the more they stay the same.) Peter learned that two members—Ananias and his wife Sapphira— were covetous deceivers. The apostles needed to confront the couple. Ananias came first. After trying to lie his way out of the charges, he dropped dead on the spot. Three hours later Peter addressed Sapphira. She too dropped dead. Leadership is not for cowards!

However, notice the ensuing response: "So great fear came upon all the church and upon all who heard these things" (Acts 5:11). The people were awestruck; I imagine the events of that day lived on, emblazed in their memories. Those two bodies bore witness of God's nature—He is holy, and He calls His people to holiness. But notice something else. Peter emerged unscathed by the membership. No biblical evidence exists that he suffered any backlash or heard any derogatory remarks about this event.

Unbelievable! Why? A similar event today would prompt enormous repercussions. At the very least I can envision a mass exodus, a significant drop in offerings, and a heated attempt to remove Peter from office. Slander and gossip would prevail as people dragged Peter's character through the mud. I can almost hear the tongues clucking: "Such nerve! Did Peter forget he denied Jesus? Hypocrite! What he did to that couple was disgraceful! All they were trying to do was give an offering—and Peter killed them! He's the greedy one! I'm leaving this church!"

Alas, church discipline is never easy, but it's necessary. Receive it and grow. Remember Proverbs 3:12 says the Lord corrects those He loves.

5. Reciprocating

As a pastor's wife, over the years I have heard my share of church complaints. Younger people often complain that seniors operate under a double standard. While they expect to be treated a certain way, they don't reciprocate (failing to return kindness and respect, for example). Even something seniors might dismiss as insignificant, like remembering a young person's name, is important. If a young person knows your name, you ought to know theirs, no matter how old you are.

In the long run, the church belongs to God, who is her ultimate sustainer. He determines whether a congregation will survive or close its doors. So be encouraged, and pray without ceasing! The universal church will prevail, no matter what happens on the local level. However, if membership is dwindling at your location, make sure that the habits of stodgy old people aren't behind the decline.

SOCIAL NETWORKS

Nearly every aspect of life—work, worship, recreation—links us to others. Humans are social creatures; our very survival depends on connections. Surely many of the living beings God created exist and even reproduce in isolation. Not mankind, His special handiwork. We thrive on relationships. Outside of reproduction, social ties establish our identity and culture: they are the center of holidays, anniversaries, and the way we celebrate life's major transitions. Though they come in many forms, each kind of relationship plays a distinct role:

- Intimate connections to a spouse or someone close who affirms us and gives us emotional support.

- Relationships with family members and friends provide a source of enjoyment. We also gain tangible support, such as help with difficult tasks, transportation, or finances.

- More casual connections from the workplace, neighborhood, and church instill a sense of belonging and confirm that our purpose extends beyond ourselves.

Because relationships are so fundamental, it should come as no surprise that they have a significant effect on physical and mental well-being. Flesh-and-blood social networks play a key role—either positive or negative—in vitality and longevity, especially as we age. The National Health and Nutrition Examination Survey found that the quality of relationships even changes our *perception* of health. Of the seniors polled, those who felt their support system was inadequate were twice as likely to classify themselves as having poor health, compared to those who were content with their social ties.[3]

BIBLICAL INSIGHTS

Now the two of them went until they came to Bethlehem. And it happened, when they had come to Bethlehem, that all the city was excited because of them; and the women said, "Is this Naomi?" But she said to them, "Do not call me Naomi; call me Mara, for the Almighty has dealt very bitterly with me. I went out full, and the LORD has brought me home again empty. Why do you call me Naomi, since the LORD has testified against me, and the Almighty has afflicted me?" So Naomi returned, and Ruth the Moabitess her daughter-in-law with her, who returned from the country of Moab. Now they came to Bethlehem at the beginning of barley harvest."

—RUTH 1:19–22

This account is one of the most tender in the Bible. One of its many lessons relates to the impact of relationships on health—in Naomi's case, mental health in particular.

For the sake of background for those not familiar with the story, Naomi, her husband, and her two sons travelled to Moab to escape a famine. While there, her sons married two Moabite girls named Ruth and Orpah. Then calamity struck. Her husband and sons died, leaving Naomi a widow in an era when that spelled helplessness.

When Naomi decided to return to her hometown of Bethlehem, only Ruth accompanied her, meaning Naomi's social network quickly dwindled from five to one.

Even though Ruth was devoted and caring, her kindness did not minimize Naomi's loss. She expressed her grief in stark terms, insisting instead of Naomi (meaning pleasant) others call her Mara (meaning bitter). In her estimation, the latter more suitably described what she had endured, and who she had become.

This passage marks the end of chapter 1, clearly a low point in Naomi's life. Yet chapter 2 marks the turning point. Although the first chapter ends in a tone of sorrow, the next begins with the words, "There was a relative..." Thus starts the healing process where Naomi becomes *pleasant* again. Her spirit of bitterness lifts and ushers in a fresh season of hope. Her social network—relatives, friends, and community—provided the keys to restoration. Thank God for the healing power of relationships!

Without a doubt, positive relationships are beneficial to our health. Yet good relationships don't happen by chance; they require nurturing and development. So do family connections. Mutual DNA makes for ties, but not enough to make ties that thrive! One attribute of healthy relationships is a balance in the "give and take" dynamic. Depending on the circumstances, sometimes you're the one giving the most; at other times you're receiving. But it should average out in the long run. (If it doesn't, that may be a sign you're in an *unhealthy* relationship.)

As discussed previously, giving helps to keep us well. Whatever the circumstances, it is always better to give than to receive. One advantage to growing older is how it brings more opportunities to give. When our kids become independent, and especially after we retire, we can enjoy the blessing of "free time." But free time ought not to be "me time"—at least not all of it! Set aside time to serve others. Not only do acts of giving help seal relationships, but they carry the bonus of a positive impact on our health and well-being.

I know lots of seniors. Lots. Trust me when I say that those who are aging gracefully have a few things in common, one of which is the habit of giving. I've been immensely blessed by the example set by the many "serving seniors" I know, particularly at our church:

- My mother-in-law has been the administrator of our Christian Education Department for years. She selects the curricula, creates the monthly schedule, and helps train those who teach. Recently she decided to pursue her master's degree in theology, just so she is better equipped.

- Our church's food pantry serves thousands of needy families each year. Our volunteer roster includes dozens of names, but most can only help as time permits. Thankfully we have a core group of people who are present on a consistent basis. All are seniors. Along with food, they give smiles and much-needed words of encouragement.

- My mother and a few other seniors regularly visit a nursing home in our community to share with residents. When our church started a Girl Scout troop, my mother was one of the first to volunteer.

I could go on listing many charitable deeds seniors perform. However, I am sorry to say I also know plenty who are not so generous. They usually must be *asked* to serve. And, while not inclined to give, they expect to receive (remember that unhealthy give-and-take dynamic). A self-centered mind-set makes for a stagnant, dissatisfied life. This is why Solomon wrote, "The generous soul will be made rich, and he who waters will also be watered himself" (Prov. 11:25). If you are feeling discontented, practice giving. If you need a refreshing, serve others and get replenished.

BIBLICAL INSIGHTS

Now when Jesus had come into Peter's house, He saw his wife's mother lying sick with a fever. So He touched her hand, and the fever left her. And she arose and served them.

—MATTHEW 8:14–15

Three of the four Gospel writers relate the story of Peter's sick mother-in-law. Mark's and Luke's accounts include "immediately" to describe how quickly she was healed. Jesus truly is the Great Physician! Something else happened quickly: Peter's mother-in-law "arose and served them." What motivated her? Was it just the expectation of women in that culture? Was it part of her personality, like Jesus's friend Martha? Or did she serve out of gratitude, thankful to be whole again? All three may have played a role. Whatever the motivation, there's a lesson to be gleaned from her story: serving others comes naturally to those who've been touched by the Master.

People generous by nature are more likely to have strong, diverse social networks. I have already made the point that it is better to give than to receive. By all means, don't consider this a mere cliché. The concept of giving and receiving encompasses much more. It is a spiritual law with a "word picture" in the natural realm. Giving and receiving parallels sowing and reaping. The former is spiritual, the latter is natural—but both are real! Paul speaks to this in Galatians: "Do not be deceived, God is not mocked; for whatever a man sows, that he will also reap" (Gal. 6:7).

When it comes to aging, I've seen this spiritual law come to pass in pleasant and painful ways. The many hats I wear bring me in contact with many seniors. I'm a physician, a pastor's wife, and I serve on the board of directors for Covenant Retirement Communities—one of the nation's largest continuing care retirement communities. In these capacities, I've seen various aspects of aging, and have been part of many death and dying experiences. Unfortunately, some people spend their final days (or years) alone. Not just in solitude, but lonely, isolated, and even neglected. It is heartbreaking.

When this happens, we often tend to blame the family, especially the children. However, such a view may mean we don't know the whole story. Now, I am in no way justifying elder neglect! As believers we are called to show compassion to the "least of these" (Matt. 25:45), which includes elderly men and women with little social support. Such acts of mercy are the same as ministering to Jesus Himself. What I mean by "the whole story" is this: the law of sowing and reaping will reveal itself in the long run.

I have seen adult children care for aging parents who require round-the-clock assistance and supervision. They meet their parents' profound needs without complaint. But I have also observed older men and women with relatively minor needs who can't depend on anyone. They strain to find help for such a minor task as a trip to the grocery store.

Why the difference in these two contrasting pictures? Obviously at times the problem rests with self-centered, hard-hearted children. As I noted earlier, anyone can give birth to a fool! Yet at other times, it is spiritual laws at work. Don't be deceived: we cannot reap a harvest where we haven't planted seed. If we want a bounty of caring relationships in our latter years, we must sow the right seeds in our former years. When we sow good seed into the lives of others, the harvest is manifested in actions and attitudes. The family members and friends are pleased, even honored, to care for elderly people who have invested in their lives. When they sow little, others render care like any other "obligation." It becomes a chore rather than a deed from a loving heart.

BIBLICAL INSIGHTS

Her children rise up and call her blessed.
—Proverbs 31:28

These words describe a woman whose life epitomized sacrifice. Though the Bible doesn't give her name, I have heard her called "the Virtuous Woman," "the Wife of Noble Character," and "the Proverbs 31 Woman." She is hard working and possesses business savvy, but you may have missed her role as a caregiver. Now, there is no mention of her having elderly parents. But in describing a caregiver, Cheryl Woodson, MD, a geriatrician and author of *To Survive Caregiving*, says "If you are responsible for any care given to a person who cannot meet all of his or her own needs, you are a caregiver."[4] I think those words aptly describe the Virtuous Woman. So we can add "caregiver" to her long list of positive attributes.

While this may sound like a stretch to some, Proverbs chapter 31 lists examples of how she met the needs of her husband, servants, and children. She invested in the *lives* of people in her *life*. She reaped a great harvest, none better than her children calling her blessed. The Bible does not reveal how long she lived or how she spent her senior years. Verse 25 says "she shall rejoice in time to come"—not much information to go on. But my spiritual imagination tells me that in older years she enjoyed the benefits of a plentiful social network. I doubt she ever felt alone or forsaken. To do so would violate a spiritual law: seeds of kindness yield the fruit of compassion.

CAREGIVING

Over the course of a lifetime, most people will come face-to-face with this challenging side of life—either as providers or recipients. Sometimes the need for assistance comes in the blink of an eye. With a stroke, a person can go from self-sufficiency to dependency in minutes. Yet in other situations (particularly dementia), the shift is gradual and the amount of help required increases gradually. Within this transition are "gray zones" where the appropriate level of care is not always crystal clear.

One of my delightful elderly patients can attest to this. At ninety, Mrs. P is in remarkably good health, physically and mentally. She lives independently and still drives. What little assistance she needs comes from her senior-age daughters. Of course they are concerned about her well-being and check on her daily by phone or in person. At a recent appointment, she told me about an unsettling episode. Though we laughed about it, it speaks to the confusion that arises from aging transitions, particularly with respect to caregiving.

On the Sunday before her appointment, Mrs. P spoke to her daughter early in the morning. At the time, she intended to spend the day at home rather than attend church. An hour or so later, she changed her mind, got dressed, and left—without calling her daughter to tell her. Afterwards, Mrs. P went to lunch with a friend, unaware that her daughter had phoned again after she left for church. Of course, Mrs. P didn't answer. And like many older seniors, she doesn't use a cell phone.

Over the next few hours her daughter called several times. Finally she stopped by the apartment. Not surprisingly, no one answered. Because it was the weekend, the maintenance person wasn't there to unlock the door. So her daughter called the fire department. When Mrs. P arrived home, she found her door removed from the hinges. Inside stood her daughters and two firefighters.

Mrs. P had mixed emotions about the misunderstanding. While grateful to see such concern, she was nevertheless perturbed—even angry. She didn't understand her daughter's reaction, especially since they had just spoken. Nor did she appreciate the insulting reprimand over how she ought to "check in" before leaving her home. In her view, her daughter treated her like a child instead of the mother. This gives a good (albeit dramatic) example of how the dynamics of relationships change, and care responsibilities shift as children become providers and parents the recipients.

Certainly Mrs. P symbolizes graceful aging. She is even atypical, since most nonagenarians require far more help. However, she *is* typical with respect to who provides needed assistance. It most often comes from family members, usually the children. About 90 percent of long-term, in-home care adults need comes from relatives. They are usually not members of the health care profession and typically don't receive compensation. Indeed, the numbers are staggering. In 2009 approximately 43.5 million people served as unpaid family caregivers to someone older than fifty[5]—figures expected to rise as the overall population ages.

Caregiving is not just for the elderly, even though a large proportion of recipients are older. And even among adults, it comes in any number of variations. Consider these real-life situations from my medical practice:

- An eighty-year-old woman and her sixty-year-old daughter have lived together for years. The mother is able to care for herself, but the daughter still did all the errands, cooking, and cleaning. The daughter had a stroke, which left her paralyzed on one side of her body. The mother maintains their home and is her daughter's primary caregiver.

- A woman in her middle fifties has a younger sister with Down's syndrome. Their eighty-four-year-old mother has been her younger sister's primary caregiver since birth. In recent years, the mother developed Parkinson's disease and experienced significant decline in cognitive functions. The older sister moved them both into her home and is now their primary caregiver.

- Several years ago, complications during a surgical procedure left a sixty-seven-year-old man with blindness. A registered nurse, his wife had been his primary caregiver, but recently suffered a stroke, leaving her with significant physical deficits. Although she has recovered some functions, their married daughter (who has small children) has assumed the role of their primary caregiver.

The reality is this: today, stories like these are common. Most internists I know could match them and share more complex scenarios from their practices. Without a doubt, long-term caregiving—in all its varied aspects—is the norm. And it can be utterly exhausting. Yet it would be biased to focus attention on the negative aspects without including a look at the positive.

Benefits of caregiving

We've already discussed the advantages that come from putting the needs of others first. When the heart of the caregiver is sacrificial, purges feelings of frustration (which lead to anger), and casts away any inclination toward self-pity, people position themselves to receive blessings. Certainly there are tangible rewards, particularly if the position includes financial compensation. However, don't overlook the many intangible benefits:

- *Caregiving reminds us of the value of life.* My husband and I recently attended a conference on eugenics and bioethics hosted by the Christian Medical and Dental Association. The speaker, Dr. Christopher Hook, is an associate professor of medicine at Mayo Clinic and chairperson of the Mayo Enterprise Ethics Committee. Participants engaged in an eye-opening discussion, delving into a host of subjects, including genetic engineering, Nazism, racism, and a detailed history of Planned Parenthood. The conference's underlying theme stuck with me: life is valuable. When done in the right spirit, caregiving affords a priceless opportunity to see the inherent value of every life—irrespective of age, illness, or disability.

- *Caregiving is biblical.* A reliable sign of personal growth, whether spiritual or otherwise, is a willingness to place responsibilities before longings. The mature person knows the difference between "wants" and "needs." As we draw closer to God, something miraculous happens—our desires line up with His. And His desires are spelled out in His Word, including our responsibility to care for others. As James says, "Pure and undefiled religion before God and the Father is this: to visit orphans and widows in their trouble..." (James 1:27). When our motivation is obedience to God, the most burdensome tasks become bearable, even joyful.

• *Caregiving strengthens ties and makes for lasting memories.* When my father's health declined, my sisters and I faced the reality of caregiving for the first time. All four of us are Boomers, and two of us are "sandwiched" (which we'll discuss in the next section). Was it stressful? Without a doubt. Were there times of conflict? Several. How did it feel? Like riding an emotional roller coaster. But did the good outweigh the bad? Absolutely. We were blessed through the entire experience. Each moment spent with Dad created priceless memories for us, his grandchildren, and great-grandchildren. The times we shared drew us closer to each other. Yes it was draining on all fronts—physically, mentally, and emotionally—but we wouldn't trade the experience for the world.

The burden of caregiving

While serving as a caregiver is a blessing, it is still a tremendous burden. One survey conducted on caregivers measured the time spent providing care and the recipient's level of dependency. Based on the results, 32 percent of caregivers classified their duties as "high burden," and 19 percent as "medium burden." The average caregiver spends about twenty hours per week providing care; one in five devotes more than forty hours per week to the task.[6] This includes everything from assisting with bathing to dressing and eating, to managing medications and finances, providing transportation, and giving emotional support.

Caregiver stress is extremely common—some might say it approaches an epidemic. It is so common that health care professionals are now encouraged to assess the well-being of the person *bringing* the patient, as well as the patient. Although frequently overlooked, it is nevertheless considered a serious condition impacting both the provider of care and (indirectly) the recipient. While no specific criteria categorize the level of stress, college professor Steven H. Zarit and his colleagues propose the following definition for caregiver burden: "The extent to which caregivers perceive that caregiving has had an adverse effect on their emotional, social, financial, physical, and spiritual functioning."[7]

This speaks to the all-encompassing nature of the stress and how it can impact every aspect of life. Anyone can become overwhelmed with the responsibility of caring for someone else. Those who are especially susceptible to caregiver burden are more likely to have the following characteristics:

- Female gender
- Low educational level
- Depression
- Social isolation
- Financial strain
- Reside with the care recipient
- Spend a large number of hours providing care
- Have no choice in acting as the caregiver

In 1981 social worker Dorothy Miller coined the term "Sandwich Generation." It refers to anyone "sandwiched" between caring for two sets of people, usually parents and children. An estimated one in every eight Americans between forty and sixty is in such a situation. Of course, those numbers are bound to increase in the near future.

If you are a caregiver, especially a "sandwiched" caregiver, recognize the burden can be overwhelming. Don't ignore the stress. Instead, take whatever steps are necessary to reduce it. Tap into any resources available in your community, whether through Medicare or other insurance plans. Consider hiring someone to assist you, even if only for a few hours a week. Investigate adult day-care programs and don't be ashamed to ask for help from family members. Remember, your health is as high a priority as the recipient's. You won't be equipped to take care of another if you fall apart yourself. Finally, don't get overwhelmed with guilt if it turns out that a move to an assisted living or skilled nursing facility represents the best option.

Here are a few websites for caregivers that may help you connect with untapped resources, or at least be a source of encouragement:

- US Centers for Disease Control and Prevention: http://www.cdc.gov/aging/caregiving/resources.htm

- AARP Caregiving Resource Center: http://www.aarp .org/home-family/caregiving

- The Caregiver Action Network: http://caregiver action.org

- Family Caregiver Alliance: http://www.caregiver.org

BIBLICAL INSIGHTS

When Jesus therefore saw His mother, and the disciple whom He loved standing by, He said to His mother, "Woman, behold your son!" Then He said to the disciple, "Behold your mother!" And from that hour that disciple took her to his own home.
—JOHN 19:26–27

Jesus's life was brief, yet wonderful. He was fully human. Like all of humanity, His life included the transitions of birth and death. But as God incarnate, He was also fully divine, so His transitions were anything but ordinary. They were monumental, impacting the universe.

In the account from John, Jesus is on the brink of death. He has been charged, arrested, tried, and now hangs on a cross, prepared to take on the sins of humanity. What a glorious moment for all mankind! His sacrifice paid our debt; His suffering secured our liberty. The magnitude of this task is incomprehensible, yet it didn't cause Him to lose sight of a "minor detail." His mother would need a caregiver.

By now, Mary's husband, Joseph, had more than likely died. As her oldest son, Jesus faced the primary responsibility for her care, especially as she grew older. This passage offers two life lessons.

First, we see the importance of advance care planning. Jesus eliminates confusion by communicating His plan for Mary *before* He dies. We also see His concern for the defenseless. His transition to death would leave Mary vulnerable. She would need someone to look after her needs. This was so important to Him that He took time out to make arrangements, even in the process of saving the world.

However, don't miss the other significant element. His eye was not just on Mary. Jesus also saw John, the one who would assume the burden of caring for His mother. What a responsibility! To be primary caregiver for the woman who gave birth to the Messiah! The lesson for caregivers is this: Jesus gave this duty to His friend. If you are a caregiver, rest in the knowledge that Jesus is your friend. He sees you, and He cares.

Chapter 5

INTIMACY

I am my beloved's, and his desire is toward me.
—Song of Solomon 7:10

GOD CREATED ADAM and then gave him a job: caretaker of the Garden of Eden. In the beginning Adam lived and worked alone, but God didn't make this a permanent condition: "And the LORD God said, 'It is not good that man should be alone; I will make him a helper comparable to him'" (Gen. 2:18). Before God created Eve, though, He made sure Adam understood his plight. So He gave Adam the responsibility of naming the animals. In so doing, Adam observed the pattern for companionship. Every creature had a mate, yet these twosomes weren't identical—alike, yet different. When the ducks waddled before him, Adam must have noticed a brightly colored drake and a hen with dull feathers. Yet both had webbed feet. Very different, yet very much alike. Adam saw the same pattern with every species.

Even though Adam enjoyed a pure, divine relationship with God, *something was missing.* By the time he completed his task, Adam recognized the void in his life. Genesis 2:20 confirms this: "So Adam gave names to all cattle, to the birds of the air, and to every beast of the field. But for Adam there was not found a helper comparable to him." In the verses that follow, God creates Eve, demonstrating how He designed us for companionship and instilled a desire for intimacy within us that lasts throughout our lifetimes.

CREATED FOR INTIMACY

First, let's clarify terms. I will use *intimacy* to refer to meaningful relationships in general. Yes, the term can refer specifically to sexual intimacy, but in the generic sense it speaks to close relationships. I don't want terminology to be a source of confusion. It is in keeping with God's design that all of humanity engage in *intimate* relationships. But it is *not* in keeping with God's design that all of humanity engage in *sexual* relationships. The latter is reserved for those bonded together by the covenant of marriage.

Now that society's attitudes toward sex and senior citizens are more open, we can thank Solomon for giving us a biblical balance on the proper framework for marital intimacy. Among the many exchanges between him and his beloved is this one: "I am the rose of Sharon, and the lily of the valleys. Like a lily among thorns, so is my love among the daughters. Like an apple tree among the trees of the woods, so is my beloved among the sons. I sat down in his shade with great delight, and his fruit was sweet to my taste. He brought me to the banqueting house, and his banner over me was love" (Song of Sol. 2:1–4).

I once heard a speaker say that sexual intimacy was God's wedding gift to married couples. Although I like that analogy, I want to expand on the comparison. Unlike a toaster oven or a setting of fine china, God's wedding gift is the only one that will

- strengthen the marriage bond;

- add excitement;

- not go out of style;

- reduce stress;

- keep a smile on your face;

- help you sleep;

- not end up in a garage sale; and

- produce more God-given gifts (children!).

It brings all that and so much more—truly the gift that keeps on giving. God reveals His plan for marriage in many Bible passages, but especially in the Song of Solomon, which represents love poetry at its finest. It celebrates the harmony and bliss of holy matrimony while highlighting the joy of sexual intimacy. In the context of marriage, Scripture affirms sex as private, but not shameful. Mysterious, but not taboo. It is a facet of the supernatural union described in Genesis: "Therefore a man shall leave his father and mother and be joined to his wife, *and they shall become one flesh*" (Gen. 2:24, emphasis added).

"One flesh" speaks to procreation as well as the sexual bond. There is a time limitation on the former (we can't bear children forever), but none on the latter. The concept of "one flesh" extends throughout marriage—from a spiritual and physical perspective. Yes, the manner and frequency of sexual expression will change over time. Still, growing older does not mean we lose the desire for intimate contact.

The Baby Boomer generation changed our thinking about many stereotypes, including sexuality. In years past, society didn't readily accept the idea of sexually active older adults. People looked at sex as something for young people and considered anyone who continued to engage past their young adult life as "deviant" or "weird." Now, older adults have always had sex; it just wasn't a topic for public discussion. So for years people skirted the issue, lest one be labeled depraved. This silence extended into the doctor's office—and doctors didn't help! What patients left unsaid physicians didn't investigate. Though trained to take detailed, head-to-toe health histories, they routinely passed over the area from the midsection to the thighs.

Then along came Viagra. That medication and others like it proved instrumental in reducing the embarrassment. If a virile, handsome man in a prime-time TV ad could talk openly about bedroom difficulties, then why should anyone feel ashamed? And the commercials ventured beyond the bedroom—even the great outdoors could be a fine location for a rendezvous! The little blue pill virtually eliminated societal awkwardness. Seemingly overnight, blushing and stammering ceased. Sexuality in all its aspects, whether normal function or dysfunction, became a topic for open discussion.

This openness helped dispel myths about sexual activity and age. Consider a 2004 survey conducted by the American Association of Retired Persons. Of the 1,600 respondents, only 4 percent agreed with the statement "Sex is only for younger people." Seventy percent disagreed or strongly disagreed with the statement "I do not particularly enjoy sex."[1] Another study involving 27,500 adults over age forty had similar results. In that one, only 17 percent of women and 23 percent of men agreed with the statement that older people lose their desire for sex; 82 percent of men and 76 percent of women believed that satisfactory sex is essential for maintaining a relationship.[2] So research confirms what "older" folks have known all along—sexual expression is not limited by age.

BIBLICAL INSIGHTS

> Drink water from your own cistern, and running water from your own well. Should your fountains be dispersed abroad, streams of water in the streets? Let them be only your own, and not for strangers with you. Let your fountain be blessed, and rejoice with the wife of your youth. As a loving deer and a graceful doe, let her breasts satisfy you at all times; and always be enraptured with her love. For why should you, my son, be enraptured by an immoral woman, and be embraced in the arms of a seductress?
> —Proverbs 5:15–20

The first section of the Book of Proverbs includes Solomon's life lessons—pearls of wisdom passed on to the next generation. Over and over you find the words "my son," along with the plea to "pay attention," "receive my words," and "do not forget." The entire fifth chapter is devoted to sex, with an emphasis on the hazards of adultery. Solomon points out the perils:

- The initial "sweetness" invariably leads to suffering (5:3–4)
- It replaces honor with shame (5:9)
- It is a source of financial ruin (5:10)
- Consequences include physical disease, even death (5:11)
- It causes mental anguish and regret (5:12)
- It leads to public disgrace (5:14)

The "seductress," as Solomon calls her, is like the devil—a master of lies. She convinces those heeding her call that sex within the confines of marriage is not enough. She is a deceiver, fooling men into believing their wives can't satisfy all their sexual needs. However, Solomon knows that sex confined to the context of marriage is a blessing! And after issuing these warnings (in graphic detail), he encourages his son to stay true to the marriage covenant, to "rejoice with the wife of your youth." Adultery is devastating. If your marriage has been damaged by infidelity, I encourage you to seek professional help and the wisdom of God.

Once sex disappeared from the "taboo" list, it raised the question of what constitutes "normal," especially for older men and women. The answer is tricky; it varies from couple to couple. Keep in mind that there is no "ideal standard" for sexuality. One person's plenty is paucity for the next. Likewise, acts that cause one couple to squirm may be par for the course for another. One reason is that so many variables come into play—past experiences, expectations, cultural issues, an individual's need for connectedness, and the dynamics of the relationship. All will affect sexual activity, irrespective of age.

Needless to say, time changes everything, including the manner and frequency of sexual expression. How a couple addresses this is important, particularly if things are "out of sync." What happens when one person is willing and able, but the other person—for whatever reason—is not? Any such barriers should be assessed, not dismissed. After discussing the nature of the problem, whether physical or emotional, appropriate treatment should follow. It goes without saying that coercion, intimidation, and extramarital affairs are not acceptable solutions. Some problems, such as fatigue, stress, and overcommitment are fixable without outside intervention. Others require help from either a physician or a therapist. Of course, sexual dysfunction can be a problem at any age. However, some issues are more common in older couples. Let's examine a few.

SEXUAL DYSFUNCTION

A wide range of conditions affect sexual function. Some are gender specific; others affect men and women. Some problems occur only in certain situations, while others are universal. Some problems appear later in life; others are manifested in younger years. In general, disorders of sexual function fall into the following categories:

- Sexual desire disorders

- Sexual arousal disorders

- Orgasmic disorders

- Sexual pain disorders

- Dysfunction due to medical conditions

Undoubtedly, other variables—stress, fatigue, and relational troubles—will exacerbate all of these. I will provide a brief overview of each category, since a comprehensive summary is beyond the scope of this book. However, I encourage you to seek medical advice as appropriate.

Sexual Desire Disorders

Sexual desire disorders run the gamut from aversion to any form of sexual contact to a modest (albeit significant) decline in interest. Extreme aversion may result from a history of trauma, such as incest, rape, or other forms of sexual abuse. Milder forms of aversion often appear because of a fear of causing personal harm, or harm to the partner. Some men and women, for instance, avoid intercourse if they or their partner has heart disease. The thought of having a massive heart attack while engaging in sex is distressing enough to curtail activity—even after a cardiologist gives the OK. Additionally there are strong cultural biases in the level and expression of sexual desire, particularly for women. Cross-cultural studies have shown that the frequency of intercourse, the level of enjoyment, and the degree of inhibition varies widely based on race and ethnicity.

BIBLICAL INSIGHTS

Let him kiss me with the kisses of his mouth—for your love is better than wine.
—Song of Solomon 1:2

God designed humans in such a way that we thrive on being touched. Proof appears at birth, when newborn infants need to be cuddled to survive. Those denied skin-to-skin contact can develop a condition known as "failure to thrive." Throughout life, touching comes in many forms and varies by setting. In some, a handshake or a pat on the back may be appropriate; in other circumstances, an embrace is best. There are cultural nuances too. In some African countries men walk hand in hand as a sign of platonic friendship. You don't see that too much in America. And in some ethnic groups, everybody hugs everybody—friends and strangers alike. In mixed crowds, such expressions can unsettle folks from other races! Of course, touch sets the foundation for sexual intimacy, as seen in the kisses and hugs beautifully described in the Song of Solomon.

Yet touch, like so many of God's gifts, can be perverted. That which God created to bless is transformed into a curse when done in the wrong setting, or by the wrong person. When the sin nature prevails, this act becomes inappropriate, abusive, and depraved. Unfortunately, many people, both males and females, are the victims of sexual abuse—an offense that starts with a touch. Past sexual abuse can impact every aspect of life, particularly intimate relationships and normal sexual function. When not dealt with, the hurt can be evident into the senior years. If someone violated you, help is available and healing is possible.

We know the sex hormones, estrogen and testosterone, play a role in sexual responsiveness. What is less clear is how much the age-related decline in these hormones contributes to desire. Certainly other variables are involved. Research is ongoing in this area, especially for women. While the hormonal changes that occur over time are not pathologic per se, they are responsible for many physiological changes. In this chapter we will discuss their role in sexual function along with some of the medical issues related to midlife hormonal changes.

MENOPAUSE

Menopause is the permanent loss of the menstrual cycle. Women who have their ovaries removed surgically experience it immediately. However, in the absence of surgery, a woman enters this phase of life over a span of time, as long as five to six years. The transition begins with a progressive decline in the function of the ovaries (particularly the production of estrogen) and the regular release of eggs (ovulation). This phase, called perimenopause, lasts for several years with typical symptoms of hot flashes, night sweats, and irregular menstrual cycles. Thankfully, after the menstrual periods stop, the symptoms gradually decline.

By definition, a woman is considered postmenopausal one year after her final period. The average age is fifty-one, and is influenced by genetics and environmental factors. Mothers and daughters tend to go through menopause around the same age. Women who smoke will commonly experience it at an earlier age.

Of course, the physiological changes of menopause affect sexual function and much more! The symptoms include

- hot flashes and night sweats (also called "vasomotor symptoms");

- painful intercourse;

- changes in sexuality (libido, arousal, enjoyment, responsiveness);

- mood changes (depression, irritability, anxiety);

- sleep disturbances;

- weight gain and bloating;

- changes in cognitive function (memory, concentration);

- breast tenderness;

- nonspecific physical symptoms (fatigue, muscle aches, joint pain);

- headache;

- abnormal and irregular vaginal bleeding;

- loss of bladder control; and

- reduced quality of life, diminished sense of well-being.

Any woman who has endured menopause will agree the symptoms are broad and diverse. One of the greatest challenges is determining the culprit. How can we be sure the source of the problem is hormonal, versus one of the many nonhormonal facets of aging? And there is much overlap, which only adds to the confusion. Take insomnia, for instance. If a woman develops difficulty sleeping at mid-life, are night sweats to blame? Or are concerns like the declining health of her parents and whether she has adequate retirement savings causing her to toss and turn? Both affect sleep— the former is related to estrogen; the latter is part of life.

Menopausal symptoms are extremely common. The intensity varies from woman to woman, but nearly all will experience something, even if minimal. Some symptoms like hot flashes steadily improve and usually resolve over time. Others, particularly vaginal dryness, tend to progress. This is because the drop in estrogen reduces the amount of lubricant produced by the glands in the vulva and cervix. The genital tissue becomes thin and less elastic (a process known as "atrophy"). It also becomes dry. The end result is that intercourse may be uncomfortable, even painful.

But be encouraged! While menopause is a major change, marking the end of the stage of fertility, it does not signal the end of sexuality. Yes, the physiological changes that come with menopause affect all females to some degree. However, their effect on sexual response is highly variable. One European study found that hormones, while playing a significant role with respect to sexual desire, are definitely not the only factor. These researchers followed close to four hundred premenopausal women over the span of eight years as they transitioned into menopause. Interestingly, sexual response after menopause stemmed more from the woman's feelings for her partner and their prior level of sexual activity. Estrogen did have some effect in sexual desire, but the quality of the relationship turned out to be much more significant.

BIBLICAL INSIGHTS

Let your speech always be with grace, seasoned with salt, that you may know how you ought to answer each one.

—COLOSSIANS 4:6

To be sure, a satisfying sex life does not *make* a strong relationship. Instead, it is a *result* of a good relationship and *evidence* of its strength. Problems in the bedroom rarely start in there; all too often the culprit is communication. Effective communication begins with two things: the ability to listen, and the wisdom to say the right thing. Both are easier said than done. They require a high level of discipline, combined with a willingness to yield. Without good communication, every aspect of the relationship will suffer, including sex.

Paul addresses communication in his epistles; Colossians 4:6 is a prime example. What we say, and how we say it, ought to reflect who we are as believers. Unfortunately, we are sometimes more graceful in the way we speak to strangers than we are to our spouses. And for women in particular, the connection between speech and sex is powerful. Conversations taking place during the day—whether positive or negative—will show up in the bedroom at night. Never underestimate the power of words. Just as salt preserved food in days of old, so properly seasoned words will preserve our relationships.

Sometimes a woman assumes desire is the problem when the underlying issue is discomfort. She will avoid intercourse because it's painful. Menopause does not always cause dryness. Other medical conditions, including diabetes and autoimmune disorders, are sometimes the culprit. In addition, vaginal dryness is a potential side effect for over one hundred commonly used medications. If a woman experiences this, there are several options, starting with over-the-counter lubricants and moisturizers. They can alleviate discomfort without any long-term safety risks, and you don't need a prescription.

OVER-THE-COUNTER VAGINAL LUBRICANTS AND MOISTURIZERS

NAME	DOSING	FEATURES
K-Y Jelly	No specific recommended dose; used as needed.	Lubricant only; used at time of intercourse.
Replens	Every 3–5 days, although can be used daily	Vaginal moisturizer; recommended scheduled dosing with additional application (if needed) prior to intercourse.
Luvena Prebiotic	Every 3 days	Vaginal lubricant and moisturizer.

There are times, however, when lubricants and moisturizers don't adequately reduce discomfort. And quite often, vaginal dryness is just one of a myriad of menopausal symptoms. Since none of these products does anything with respect to hormone levels, let's take a moment to review menopause from a broader perspective than sexual function.

The symptoms of menopause, particularly the vasomotor symptoms, are treated in a number of ways. In mild cases, lifestyle modification alone—such as adding exercise, yoga, and other forms of relaxation—can provide satisfactory relief. Avoid spicy foods, alcohol, excessive sugar, and hot drinks, all of which can trigger hot flashes. Nothing beats plain common sense: wear cool clothing and pajamas, dress in layers, use a fan, and turn the thermostat down at night.

Beyond lifestyle modification, some women respond well to alternative approaches. Now, such methods as acupuncture, hypnosis, and supplements like black cohosh, St. John's wort, and red clover have had mixed results in clinical trials. Many well-designed studies didn't show any benefit beyond a placebo effect. Nevertheless, plenty of women notice a significant improvement in using them. Physicians routinely prescribe several medications for hot flashes and night sweats. The antidepressants fluoxetine, citalopram, escitalopram, and sertraline—as well as clonidine and gabapentin—all show benefits in relieving vasomotor symptoms. In 2013 the Food and Drug Administration (FDA) approved paroxetine (Brisdelle) as the first nonhormonal therapy for hot flashes. And we can expect other nonhormonal treatments to gain approval in the near future.

While these products may be worth trying, nothing relieves the symptoms of menopause as effectively as hormone therapy. It minimizes hot flashes and night sweats better than any other method, and also reverses genital atrophy and vaginal dryness. Estrogen is used as a single agent in a woman without a uterus. When a woman still has her uterus, estrogen should be combined with a progesterone to reduce the risk of uterine cancer.

However, the mere mention of "hormone therapy" brings up the question, "Is it safe?" It depends. Clearly, there are definite risks. Women using hormone therapy are more likely to develop blood clots, and it increases the incidence of stroke and breast cancer. But there are also definite benefits with respect to symptom relief, including sexual function. Without question, there are some women who should not use hormone replacement therapy under any circumstances. They include those who have had

- a previous heart attack or stroke;
- a history of blood clots (e.g., deep venous thrombosis [DVT] or pulmonary embolism [PE]);
- breast cancer or uterine cancer; or
- abnormal vaginal bleeding.

In the absence of these conditions, the decision to use hormone therapy becomes highly individualized. Talk to your health care provider to determine the risks and—after assessing the pros and cons—make an educated decision. It ultimately hinges on a woman's health history, her quality of life, and whether she believes the benefits outweigh the risks. The latter speaks to values, which are not easily measured in a clinical trial. I had a patient whose hot flashes affected her quality of life to such an extent that she was willing to assume any risk, no matter how great. She was a high-ranking executive, and at the most inopportune times a hot flash would strike—so intense the perspiration soaked through her suit, dampened her hair, and smeared her makeup. Thankfully she had a relatively low risk for complications. Still, even with a moderate risk, she was determined to put an end to being embarrassed at business meetings and "power" lunches.

Other variables that factor into the decision relate to age and timing. These are actually key determinants. This crucial link to the timing of when hormonal therapy should be initiated surfaced after doctors reassessed the data from the aforementioned Women's Health Initiative. Investigators tracked these 162,000 participants for years, gathering a wealth of information on almost every aspect of their health, including hormone replacement therapy. The results of a 2002 data analysis showed a higher risk of heart disease, stroke, breast cancer, blood clots, and gallbladder disease among estrogen users. As a result, the number of prescriptions for hormone replacement plummeted overnight, a development I remember quite well. Doctors had routinely prescribed estrogen, assuming its primary benefits were healthier hearts and stronger bones. So these results were indeed surprising.

However, five years later, doctors reanalyzed this data by factoring in the woman's age and the number of years since the onset of menopause. In the initial 2002 report, the average age was sixty-five. But in the 2007 evaluation, it became clear that the risk of hormone replacement therapy varied depending on the woman's age at the time she initiated treatment. The difference was dramatic:

- For women under sixty or within ten years of menopause: *decreased* risk of heart disease, *decreased* risk of breast cancer, *decreased* total mortality.

- For women aged sixty to seventy: no change in overall risk.

- For women over seventy: *increased* risk of heart disease, *increased* risk of stroke, *increased* risk of blood clots, *increased* total mortality.

Therefore, timing is everything when it comes to such therapy. For younger women at low risk, hormone replacement is acceptable for treating symptoms of menopause. Estrogen therapy (not combined estrogen-progesterone therapy) may actually reduce heart disease risk in younger women when initiated soon after the onset of menopause. Hormone therapy, however, is not approved for use in *preventing* diseases like heart disease, dementia, and osteoporosis. With respect to *treating* osteoporosis, it is considered a second line agent (see chapter 3).

With respect to bioidentical hormone therapy, the North American Menopause Society and the American Congress of Obstetricians and Gynecologists do not recommend custom-compounded preps because of issues related to regulatory oversight, a lack of data on safety and efficacy, and concerns regarding batch-to-batch consistency.

The following table lists several forms of hormone replacement currently available:

FDA APPROVED HORMONE REPLACEMENT THERAPY			
DRUG	**PREPARATION**	**BRAND NAMES**	**DOSING**
Conjugated Estrogens	Oral	Premarin, Cenestin, Enjuvia	Premarin: 0.3125–0.625 mg daily Cenestin, Enjuvia: 0.3–1.25 mg daily (continuously or cyclically)
	Oral Combination to treat vasomotor symptoms and osteoporosis (selective estrogen receptor modulator + conjugated estrogen)	Duavee	20 mg/0.45 mg daily
	Vaginal Cream	Premarin	0.5 g intra-vaginally twice weekly for 21 days on and 7 days off, or continuously
Esterified Estrogens	Oral	Menest	0.3–1.25 mg daily (continuously or cyclically)
Estradiol	Oral	Estrace, Femtrace	0.5–2 mg daily

FDA APPROVED HORMONE REPLACEMENT THERAPY			
DRUG	**PREPARATION**	**BRAND NAMES**	**DOSING**
Estradiol	Transdermal	Alora, Estraderm, Vivelle-Dot, Climara	1 patch (0.025–0.1 mg/day) applied to trunk or buttocks. Replace Climara weekly; replace Alora, Estraderm and Vivelle-Dot twice weekly
	Topical Gel	Divigel, Elestrin, EstroGel	Apply daily (Divigel to upper thigh; Elestrin and EstroGel to upper arm)
	Topical Emulsion Spray	Estrasorb, Evamist	Apply daily (Estrasorb to legs; Evamist to forearm)
	Vaginal Ring	Femring, Estring	Insert one ring vaginally every 3 months
	Vaginal Cream	Estrace	1 g intravaginally 1–3 times weekly for 3 weeks on, 1 week off

FDA APPROVED HORMONE REPLACEMENT THERAPY			
DRUG	**PREPARATION**	**BRAND NAMES**	**DOSING**
Estradiol	Vaginal Tablet	Vagifem	10 mcg or 25 mcg intra-vaginally twice weekly
	Intramuscular Injection	Delestrogen, Depo-Estradiol	Delestrogen: 10–20 mg every 4 weeks as needed Depo-Estra-diol: 1–5 mg every 3–4 weeks as needed
Estropipate	Oral	Ogen, Ortho-Est	0.75–6 mg daily
Conjugated Estrogen + Medroxypro-gesterone	Oral	Prempro, Premphase	Prempro: Start with lowest dose daily (0.3/1.5 mg); Prem-phase: 0.625 mg estrogens daily on days 1–14, then 0.625/5 mg daily on days 15–28

Testosterone deficiency

The concentration of testosterone gradually falls with age. For men, an experienced health writer coined the term "manopause" to describe these hormonal changes. The rate of decline is slower for men who are physically fit and in good health. Like other hormones, testosterone has multiple physiological effects. In addition to its role in a man's sexual function, testosterone also helps to maintain bone density, muscle mass, and muscle strength.

Deficiency in older men is fairly common, though the exact prevalence is unknown. One reason: accurate confirmation of the testosterone level is cumbersome. It requires two separate blood draws, which must occur early in the morning, since blood drawn late in the day does not yield a reliable measurement. The symptoms of low testosterone include fatigue, depression, loss of libido, and insomnia. Many of these symptoms are nonspecific and overlap with other medical and psychological problems.

Replacement therapy is recommended *only* for men with a confirmed deficiency. In other words, the decision to treat should be based upon the amount of testosterone measured by a blood test and not on symptoms alone. Once a man starts replacement therapy, his testosterone should be remeasured in three to six months to confirm the level has reached the normal range. The number of men currently prescribed some form of testosterone is high. Rest assured, not all of these men are deficient. Use among men age forty or older more than tripled between 2001 and 2011. One study found that 25 percent of all the men given a prescription for testosterone replacement therapy had not had their levels measured during the entire year prior to starting treatment.[3] As with many medications, pharmaceutical companies aggressively market testosterone replacement therapy to both physicians and patients. The latter is particularly effective.

Currently, testosterone replacement therapy is a hot topic in the medical and lay communities. It is commonly prescribed (sometimes appropriately; sometimes not), but the long-term risks need further investigation, particularly with respect to heart disease and other potential adverse side effects. While testosterone products have long included a warning about the increase in the risk for blood clots, labeling for cardiovascular risk has only recently become a requirement. In early 2015 the FDA mandated that all testosterone products include a warning that men using the products may be at increased risk for stroke, heart attack, and death.

This move followed an extensive evaluation of clinical trials, including two major studies published in 2013 and 2014. One suggested a higher risk for heart attack in the three months after starting a prescription. The other demonstrated a greater risk of heart attack, stroke, and death from any cause in men using testosterone compared to men who were not. However, the data was conflicting, which complicates the situation. For instance, a large study released in 2014 showed entirely different results. It showed no association between testosterone use and heart attack in more than twenty-four thousand men using the intramuscular injection form, all of whom were over sixty-five.[4] In addition, several studies show a *protective* effect where men on replacement therapy experienced *fewer* cardiovascular events. Even the mode of delivery—patch, gel, or injection—appears to play a role in overall risk.

Along with labeling changes, the FDA also emphasized that using replacement therapy for the *age-related* decline in testosterone levels has not been confirmed as beneficial. These products are approved only for treating deficiencies caused by disorders of the various organs that either produce or regulate testosterone, including the brain, testicles, and pituitary gland.

For men with confirmed deficiencies, there are several different preparations available for replacement therapy. The medications currently approved by the FDA are as follows:

FDA APPROVED TESTOSTERONE REPLACEMENT THERAPY		
PREPARATION	**BRAND NAME**	**DOSING**
ORAL	Testosterone undecanoate	Andriol	40 mg capsule, 3–4 times daily for 2–3 weeks; decrease to 1–3 capsules daily depending on response
BUCCAL	Testosterone	Striant	30 mg (1 buccal system) applied to the gums twice daily
TOPICAL	Testosterone transdermal gel	AndroGel 1.62%	40.5 mg/pump actuation; 1–4 pumps/day
	Testosterone transdermal solution	Axiron	30 mg/pump actuation; 2 pump actuations/day
	Testosterone transdermal patch	Androderm	2–4 mg/ daily applied at bedtime
INJECTION	Testosterone enanthate	Delatestryl	50–400 mg intramuscularly every 2–4 weeks
	Testosterone cypionate	DEPO-Testosterone	50–400 mg intramuscularly every 2–4 weeks

FDA APPROVED TESTOSTERONE REPLACEMENT THERAPY		
PREPARATION	**BRAND NAME**	**DOSING**
INJECTION Testosterone propionate subcutaneous pellet	Testopel	150–450 mg subcutaneously every 3–6 months

If sexual desire is unrelated to a decline in hormones, patients should pursue other causes. Seek the advice of your health care provider, who can help to determine the appropriate management.

BIBLICAL INSIGHTS

Each young woman's turn came to go in to King Ahasuerus after she had completed twelve months' preparation, according to the regulations for the women, for thus were the days of their preparation apportioned: six months with oil of myrrh, and six months with perfumes and preparations for beautifying women. Thus prepared, each young woman went to the king...

—ESTHER 2:12–13

Anyone in the health care field will attest to this truth: expect the unexpected. I recall a middle-aged couple I cared for several years ago. On one visit the wife stayed in the room with her husband because she wanted to make sure he "told me everything." He was having trouble maintaining an erection, and his wife thought he would be too embarrassed to admit it. After talking things over, I wrote him a prescription for a popular medication.

A few months later he came to a scheduled follow-up appointment alone. His first words were, "I don't need the medication you prescribed." Then he told me he never had erectile dysfunction. While his wife believed he had age-related ED, the real problem—the one causing embarrassment—was his waning sexual desire for her. While he genuinely loved her, she had "let herself go." He told me his wife devoted considerable attention to her appearance during their courtship, but after marriage she shed the effort. He didn't know how to tell her, nor the heart to do it. His admission left me dumbfounded. I awkwardly took back my prescription and changed the subject.

Here's the take-home point: ladies, men are highly tuned in to their senses! Just ask King Ahasuerus, whose wives (including Esther) spent a year on their beauty regimen before spending one night with him. No matter how long you've been together, it is still important to look good, smell good, and create an enticing atmosphere. Throw out the dingy T-shirts and invest in some nice lingerie. Light a few candles and get some scented oils. Small investments pay great dividends!

SEXUAL AROUSAL DISORDERS

Men: Erectile dysfunction

In general, men are less likely to visit a health care provider when they feel fine; some won't go even when they *aren't* feeling so well. The problem with this approach is missing crucial medical screening tests and risk assessments. For example, high cholesterol and early stages of type 2 diabetes don't make you feel bad. However, blood tests can detect them. Or take hypertension, which is called "the silent killer" for a good reason—it has no symptoms. Screening can diagnose some forms of cancer in their early stages, provided a doctor does the test while the person feels well.

Despite the benefits of receiving a periodic checkup, many men still avoid the doctor's office. Yet there is one issue that compels even those with extreme aversions to get over their hang-ups and make an appointment—erectile dysfunction, commonly known as "ED." On countless occasions, an office visit for ED has allowed me an opportunity to schedule recommended screening tests and slip in advice on nutrition, exercise, and smoking cessation. Plus, ED can represent a red flag for other problems, particularly cardiovascular disease and diabetes. Any man experiencing it should have a medical work-up to look for underlying physical conditions.

BIBLICAL INSIGHTS

> And He said, "I will certainly return to you according to the time of life, and behold, Sarah your wife shall have a son." (Sarah was listening in the tent door which was behind him.) Now Abraham and Sarah were old, well advanced in age; and Sarah had passed the age of childbearing.
> —Genesis 18:10–11

Like many biblical women, Sarah struggled with infertility. God had promised her husband, Abraham, countless descendants. Yet year after year passed with no pregnancy. How could a woman past childbearing age bear a great nation? It would take a miracle. Although Sarah laughed at the idea, God assured Abraham: "Is anything too hard for the Lord? At the appointed time I will return to you, according to the time of life, and Sarah shall have a son" (Gen. 18:14). He spoke this promise when Abraham was one hundred years old and Sarah was ninety. As promised, she bore Isaac the following year. So let's pause to take a pop quiz. What was miraculous about Isaac's conception? Was it:

A. Abraham's ability to achieve and maintain an erection?

B. Abraham having the stamina to engage in intercourse?

C. Sarah conceiving despite being in menopause?

D. All of the above?

The answer is C. Yes, the idea of a man being sexually active at the century mark is fascinating but not miraculous. In fact, Sarah died about forty years after Isaac's birth, and Abraham got remarried to a woman who bore him six more sons! The story of Abraham and his second wife, Keturah, appears in Genesis 25. Interestingly, the passage contains no mention of anything unusual (nor miraculous) about Abraham still enjoying sex, even having kids.

Now certainly every man is different. Lest I plant seeds of discouragement, let me clarify that I am not suggesting Abraham's story is the norm! My point is that growing older does not signal the end to a man's sex life. The causes of sexual dysfunction—whether medical or psychological—should be investigated rather than considered a "normal" part of aging. While the way in which intimacy is expressed might *change* over time, it does not *disappear* over time. Let's modify our thinking so that it lines up with God's plan.

One doctor defines erectile dysfunction as "the consistent or recurrent inability to attain or maintain a penile erection sufficient for sexual performance."[5] That said, it is important to distinguish normal from abnormal. Some older men assume age-related changes in erectile *function* equate to erectile *dysfunction*, but they don't. Normal aging brings with it a couple of changes: the time required to achieve an erection and the firmness of the erection. These will increase and decrease respectively. A sixty-year old man is no longer twenty. The age-related differences in performance are not pathologic, and they do not require prescription drugs. Sometimes patience, not pills, is in order!

Erectile dysfunction is extremely common, affecting half of men ages forty to seventy. Its prevalence increases with age, in part because many of the medical conditions associated with ED appear more frequently in older men. Diabetes in particular greatly increases the risk. Nearly 95 percent of diabetic men over age seventy have ED.[6]

Many factors contribute to erectile dysfunction. While it is appropriate to screen for medical conditions, not all ED indicates underlying disease. It is also important to recognize that testosterone deficiency and erectile dysfunction are two different conditions (though the marketing for testosterone replacement therapy suggests otherwise). Some causes of erectile dysfunction include

- arteriosclerosis (i.e., "blocked arteries"; hence the connection to heart disease);

- diabetes;

- smoking;

- neurological diseases or other forms of nerve damage;

- prostate enlargement;

- prior history of trauma, surgery, or radiation therapy to the pelvic area;

- alcohol and drug abuse;

- hormone imbalances;

- medication side effect (common culprits are some antihypertensive agents, anxiety medications, antihistamines, antidepressants, muscle relaxants, and various pain medications);

- psychological and emotional problems (e.g., depression, anxiety, low self-esteem, performance anxiety);

- social problems (e.g., work-related stress); and

- relationship difficulties.

Treatment for erectile dysfunction should begin with lifestyle modification. Smoking cessation is extremely important. For some men, ED provides a greater incentive to quit than the risk of emphysema and lung cancer combined! Men with obesity and a sedentary lifestyle should address that problem. Those who maintain a normal body weight and are physically fit do not experience nearly as much ED, and lower their risk for medical conditions associated with ED. If side effects from medications are the cause, let your doctor know. Usually other drugs can be prescribed you can better tolerate. Men should be screened for depression and other mental health disorders as these are commonly associated with erectile dysfunction.

The most commonly prescribed of several treatment options is oral medications. In addition, there is vacuum therapy, pellets, penile injections, and implants. The category of medications known as phosphodiesterase inhibitors have revolutionized the treatment for ED. Keep in mind, these drugs do not enhance the libido, even though commercials suggest otherwise. None should be used by men taking nitrates; men prescribed α-blocker drugs should not use vardenafil or tadalafil. The following table lists the currently available medications for erectile dysfunction:

FDA APPROVED THERAPY FOR ERECTILE DYSFUNCTION			
CLASS	**CHEMICAL NAME**	**BRAND NAME**	**DOSING**
Phosphodi-esterase type 5 Inhibitors	Sildenafil (oral)	Viagra	25, 50, or 100 mg taken 1 hour before sexual activity.
	Tadalafil (oral)	Cialis	5, 10, or 20 mg taken 1 hour before sexual activity; alternately 2.5 or 5 mg taken daily at the same time each day.

FDA APPROVED THERAPY FOR ERECTILE DYSFUNCTION			
CLASS	**CHEMICAL NAME**	**BRAND NAME**	**DOSING**
Phosphodi-esterase type 5 Inhibitors	Vardenafil (oral)	Levitra, Staxyn	5, 10, or 20 mg taken 1 hour before sexual activity; alter-nately 2.5 or 5 mg taken daily at the same time each day.
	Avanafil (oral)	Stendra	100 mg taken at least 30 minutes before sexual activity.
Prosta-glandin E1	Alprostadil (intraure-thrally, intra-cavernously)	Caverject, Edex, Muse	Caverject, Edex: initially inject 2.5 mcg, may titrate up to 40 mcg (Edex) or 60 mcg (Caverject) up to 3 times weekly. Muse: initially insert 125 or 250 mcg intraurethrally. Maximum 2 administra-tions daily.

Women: Desire and arousal

Clearly, by now, the take-home point is evident: a wide variety of issues impact sexuality. Physiology, psychology, culture, and rela-tionships all play a role. Some of the *physical* problems that surface with age can be entirely prevented by following a healthy lifestyle during the younger years. Others may not be preventable but are amenable to treatment. Of course, the mental and emotional aspects of sexuality—issues like depression, fatigue, stress, and the quality of the relationship—must be teased out and addressed appropriately. At times this may require individual or couples therapy. For both men and women, several common medications can lower the libido including drugs used to treat pain, depression, and heart disease. Switching to a different medication or an alternative form of therapy may suffice in solving the problem.

Particularly for women, decreased interest and diminished arousal are often related to multiple issues. We have covered the problem of vaginal discomfort and dryness, which are common when estrogen levels decline at menopause. But estrogen is not the only hormone that diminishes during this time in a woman's life. Testosterone levels fall as well.

Although typically considered a "male" hormone, the female body produces testosterone too. Research now confirms that it plays a key role in a woman's sexual response. Desire, arousal, orgasm, pleasure, responsiveness, and even self-image are all influenced by testosterone. Yet the data also points out the quality of the relationship and psychosocial issues play a far more significant role in a woman's sexual response.

Questions remain regarding the best approach for treating women with low levels of sexual interest, desire, and arousal. Testosterone therapy has proven benefits, and transdermal formulas are often prescribed. At this writing, however, treating women in the US is considered "off label" as it has only been approved in some overseas countries.

When testosterone is prescribed for women with sexual dysfunction, the Endocrine Society Task Force recommends the following:

- Begin with a three- to six-month trial in postmenopausal women who have no obvious risks for using testosterone.

- Measure testosterone levels before starting therapy and again in three to six weeks.

- Stop therapy at six months if a woman had shown no significant benefit.

- For women who do respond, check testosterone levels every six months.

There are currently no long-term studies confirming the safety of testosterone use in women. Potential risks include abnormalities in liver function, a decrease in the HDL ("good") cholesterol, acne, excessive facial hair growth, male-pattern hair loss, and worsening control of hypertension and heart disease.

Not surprisingly, research in this area is active. Clinical trials are ongoing, and new medications are in the process of being developed. Some, such as sildenafil (Viagra), have not shown much benefit in women. In 2015 an advisory committee recommended the FDA approve the drug flibanserin for treating low sexual desire in women, provided the labeling include detailed warnings of its side effects. On two previous occasions the committee refused a recommendation because studies failed to show an effect much better than placebo. At this writing flibanserin (which will be marketed under the name "Addyi") is awaiting a final decision from the FDA. The side effects include dizziness, fainting, and accidental injuries along with significant interactions with other medications.

Orgasmic disorders

Some people with orgasmic disorders have difficulty in reaching an orgasm, seen with a delay or the total absence of attaining an orgasm. Others achieve orgasm prematurely. A side effect of some common medications, particularly drugs used to treat depression and anxiety, can be delayed orgasm. When this is the case, changing to a different medication usually solves the problem. Trouble reaching orgasm is also seen in cases of sexual trauma or abuse.

Premature ejaculation is the opposite problem, but still falls into the category of orgasmic disorders. It is considered the most common sexual dysfunction in men, including older men. Some studies estimate the prevalence in seniors to be as high as 40 percent. Premature ejaculation is treated with the same medications that have delayed orgasm as a side effect. So a troubling side effect for one person turns out to be therapeutic for the next.

Sexual pain disorders

Some women experience pain with intercourse because of spasms occurring at the entry of the vagina when attempting intercourse. This condition is known as "vaginismus." The triggers for spasm are nonspecific—even an attempt to insert a tampon or a speculum for a Pap smear can cause severe pain. This condition occurs in women of all ages. We previously discussed one of the more common causes of painful intercourse, specifically in older women, which is the vaginal dryness and atrophy associated with menopause. Lubricants and hormonal therapy have been available for years, but a newer medication is available. Ospemifene is not a hormone but has an effect similar to estrogen on the vulva and vaginal tissue. Even though it is not estrogen, it has some of the same hormonal side effects. As such, it comes with a "Black Box" warning detailing potential risks.

Another cause of painful intercourse in women is a condition known as "vulvodynia." This is a condition seen in women of all ages. The symptoms are significant discomfort during sex, particularly a burning pain, lasting over three months, with no obvious cause. The diagnosis is one of exclusion—it's made only when a workup for other sources proves negative. Vulvodynia is two to three times more likely to occur in women with other chronic pain conditions, such as fibromyalgia, irritable bowel syndrome, and interstitial cystitis. Sexual pain disorders may require specialty care to delineate the cause. An evaluation by a gynecologist, urologist, neurologist, or a psychiatrist may be appropriate.

DYSFUNCTION DUE TO MEDICAL CONDITIONS

A healthy lifestyle preserves overall health, including sexual health. Certainly some medical conditions have a direct effect on the ability to engage in sexual activity. Cardiovascular disease, chronic obstructive pulmonary disease (COPD), arthritis, and obesity are just a few of the conditions that have a negative impact. In all things, including sexuality, a healthy lifestyle is vitally important. You are never too old to benefit from the following:

- A nutritious diet
- Adequate physical activity
- Smoking cessation
- Maintaining a healthy body weight
- Using alcohol in moderation
- Getting enough sleep

Likewise, we cannot ignore the importance of mental health. Depression, anxiety, and other psychiatric disorders (along with their treatment) can adversely affect libido and sexual performance.

Finally even if a person is blessed with perfect physical and mental health, and even if menopause and "manopause" are progressing uneventfully, there are still aspects of middle age that can adversely affect sex life. This is especially the case for those who are in the "Sandwich Generation." Those with elderly parents *and* teenagers to look after, while juggling those responsibilities with a stressful job, face tremendous demands on their time and energy. In such an environment, sex can sink lower on the priority list. Although this scenario is common, it is not the norm for graceful aging.

BIBLICAL INSIGHTS

Then they rose early in the morning and worshiped before the LORD, and returned and came to their

> house at Ramah. And Elkanah knew Hannah his
> wife, and the LORD remembered her.
>
> —1 SAMUEL 1:19

Since language is not stagnant, many words' definitions change over time. And the essence of a word's meaning is sometimes lost when interpreted from one dialect to another. Take the word *knew*, used in this verse and many other Bible passages. Its ancient meaning is quite different from modern usage. In the days of the writing of 1 Samuel, to "know" someone referred to sexual intercourse. That is a huge translational change! We all "know" lots of people, but hopefully we don't "know" them in the biblical sense.

As a marriage matures, all too often the challenges and commitments of life can impact a couple's quality time. When that happens, the spouses we "know" get placed on the back burner, leaving little time to "know" them. That is not good, nor is it God's plan for marriage. The solution comes from systematically and deliberately spending time together. Here are a few suggestions:

- Block out a slot on your weekly schedule.

- Revisit and revise your priorities.

- Don't just talk about date night; put it on your calendar.

- Squeeze in a lunch between your company's conference call and a child's soccer practice.

- Even though you have a home—get a hotel room!

If your marriage is getting stagnant, make a point of getting reacquainted. You won't regret the time spent getting to know each other—in every sense of the word!

CONTRACEPTION

Unlike menopause, when conception is no longer possible (hence, the miracle with Sarah), women in perimenopause remain fertile and still able to conceive. Granted, pregnancy is not as likely during this time of life as it is in a woman's younger years, but it happens. Half of all pregnancies in women over forty are unplanned. Many of these women assumed they were no longer fertile because of age, or their irregular menstrual cycles and hot flashes. I have heard dozens of stories from women who skipped a period, assumed it was perimenopause, and learned this happened because of a baby. What a surprise! Although children are a blessing at any age, suffice it to say that contraception remains an issue up until menopause.

BIBLICAL INSIGHTS

And Judah said to Onan, "Go in to your brother's wife and marry her, and raise up an heir to your brother." But Onan knew that the heir would not be his; and it came to pass, when he went in to his brother's wife, that he emitted on the ground, lest he should give an heir to his brother. And the thing which he did displeased the LORD; therefore He killed him also.

—GENESIS 38:8–10

Views on contraception vary widely among Christians. Some believe any form of contraception contradicts God's instruction to be fruitful, multiply, and fill the earth. Others believe that since the mandates to Adam and Noah came during a period of sparse population, it shouldn't be considered an everlasting, universal law. To further complicate matters, the Bible is somewhat vague. We can infer, but don't see specific instructions. Placing the directives to Adam and Noah aside, rest assured people practiced birth control during biblical times. They didn't have highly effective methods like today's pills, patches, devices, and injections. But knowing semen was necessary for conception, they did what they knew.

In this passage Judah's son, Onan, practiced "coitus interruptus," also called "withdrawal." While God killed him, don't let Onan's experience scare you! God didn't punish him for using birth control, but because he refused to follow divine instructions. In that culture, a childless widow was to be impregnated by her deceased husband's brother. Centuries later, Moses gave specific instructions on this practice of levirate marriages (Deut. 25:5–10). So while Onan learned a hard lesson, his story is not "proof" that God opposes contraception.

Birth control methods are essentially the same for younger couples as they are for older ones. They fall into the following categories:

- Mechanical barriers (male condom, female condom, cervical cap, diaphragm, spermicidal agents)

- Sterilization (tubal ligation, vasectomy)

- Intrauterine devices

- Periodic abstinence (natural family planning, coitus interruptus)

- Hormonal (pills, implants, injections, patches, vaginal rings)

Male condoms are the most common method of barrier contraception. With proper use, condoms are fairly effective, with an annual failure rate of 3 percent. They are readily available and inexpensive. The other barrier methods are not as convenient. The female condom is cumbersome to insert (less than 1 percent of women use one), and the diaphragm and cervical cap require a visit to a health care professional for fitting.

Sterilization is highly effective but—at least for women—is not usually considered a practical option during perimenopausal years. Most gynecologists would not subject a woman to the risks of a surgical procedure with other safe forms of birth control available and menopause right around the corner. Vasectomy, however, is a reasonable option. It is safer and more effective than female sterilization, with a failure rate of only one-tenth of one percent. It is a quick outpatient procedure, usually performed under local anesthesia in five to ten minutes.

Intrauterine devices (IUDs) are an effective and safe form of birth control. Though popular in Europe, they are still not common in the United States, where less than 2 percent of women use them. This stems from a scare back in the 1970s, when regulators pulled the Dalkon Shield IUD from the market because of complications—some fatal. The IUDs on the market today are safe, convenient, and provide years of contraception.

Most couples who choose natural forms of contraception do so because of religious or cultural beliefs. They are not especially reliable methods. Coitus interruptus is entirely dependent on the man's capacity to withdraw prior to ejaculation, with a failure rate of nearly 20 percent per year. Natural family planning involves predicting the time of ovulation, and avoiding intercourse just before and after the release of the egg. Effectiveness, then, depends on a regular menstrual cycle, which is not the case during the perimenopausal years.

Oral contraceptives have been around for more than fifty years. Other forms of hormonal contraception, such as the patch and vaginal ring, have appeared in more recent years. Early forms of birth control pills contained a fairly high amount of estrogen. Today's formulas contain a combination of estrogen and progestin, with a lower dose of estrogen in an effort to improve safety. The risk of adverse side effects is related to the estrogen component. They are more frequent with higher doses of estrogen in older women, and in the presence of smoking and other medical conditions. These include the following:

- *Blood clots.* Estrogen has the capacity to activate the body's blood clotting system. This complication is not as common with low doses. Some women are at a greater risk, particularly those who smoke, are overweight or obese, or who have diabetes, hypertension, or cardiovascular disease.

- *Hypertension.* This complication is definitely dose dependent. As many as 5 percent of women using the older, high-dose pills experienced elevations in blood pressure. But even though the low-dose formulas have a minimal effect, close surveillance of blood pressure is recommended for any woman using hormonal contraceptives.

- *Cardiovascular disease.* Some studies have shown an increased risk of heart attack and stroke, but participants also had other risks for heart disease like hypertension, diabetes, obesity, and smoking.

More and more women in their late forties and fifties are using estrogen-containing oral contraceptive pills. Of course there are safety concerns, especially since those conditions associated with an increased risk—hypertension, diabetes, and obesity—become more prevalent with age. Pills containing progestin only and no estrogen (also called "minipills") are an alternative for women at increased risk for estrogen-related complications.

Do all perimenopausal women using estrogen-containing contraceptives need to switch to non-estrogen formulas? Not necessarily. Older women who are healthy, have a normal body weight, and do not smoke have a fairly low risk for complications with low-dose estrogen pills, even when their use is continued up to menopause. For women who *do not* fit this profile (and given the high prevalence of obesity and diabetes, the majority of women in the United States do not), it is best to switch to a progestin-only formula or use a nonhormonal form of birth control like condoms or an IUD. The American Congress of Obstetrics and Gynecology (ACOG) and the World Health Organization (WHO) have issued the following guidelines. Notice that the World Health Organization's recommendations are more stringent than the American Congress of Obstetrics Gynecology guidelines. It is important to discuss overall risks with a health care professional to determine your own risk-to-benefit profile.

GUIDELINES REGARDING USE OF COMBINATION ESTROGEN-PROGESTIN CONTRACEPTIVES (PILLS, PATCHES, VAGINAL RING) IN WOMEN 35 YEARS OF AGE AND OLDER		
VARIABLE	**ACOG GUIDELINES**	**WHO GUIDELINES**
Obesity	Progestin only or IUD may be safer	Benefits usually outweigh risks
Smoking	Progestin only or IUD should be used	Risk unacceptable
Hypertension	Progestin only or IUD should be used	Risk unacceptable
Diabetes	Progestin only or IUD should be used	Risk unacceptable

VARIABLE	ACOG GUIDELINES	WHO GUIDELINES
None of the above risks	Healthy nonsmoking women doing well on a combination contraceptive can continue their method until age 50–55 years, after weighing the risks and benefits.	For women ≥40 years, the risk of cardiovascular disease increases with age and may also increase with use of combined hormonal contraceptives. In the absence of other adverse clinical conditions, combined hormonal contraceptives may be used until menopause.

The take-home point is this: a woman has the potential to become pregnant until she reaches menopause. As such, she should use effective contraception to avoid unintended pregnancy. The choice of contraception is unique to the individual and to the couple, and is based on both medical and nonmedical variables. Smoking cessation and maintaining a normal body weight are always ideal but of particular importance with respect to hormonal contraceptives. If you select a hormonal form of contraception, regular medical follow-up is advised to monitor things like blood pressure, and to determine when they should be discontinued.

Chapter 6

LOSS, CONTROL, AND HOPE

What is man that You are mindful of him, and
the son of man that You visit him?

—Psalm 8:4

URING MY CHILDHOOD in the 1960s and '70s, my parents hosted bridge parties in rotation with a few other couples. They would eat and socialize as they played cards. Predictably, these chats would touch on the "new look" of a guest—often a man who wore something out of the ordinary or tried to hide his receding hairline under a thick toupée. Of course, my sisters and I had a hard time stifling our giggles. What a challenge for kids! Afterward, when my parents rehashed the evening, I would hear them toss around the term "midlife crisis." Sometimes their conversation related to trivial topics, like bell bottoms and toupees. However, they also reflected on such serious matters as adultery, divorce, and broken homes.

DEFINING A "MIDLIFE CRISIS"

Psychologist Elliot Jacques coined the term "midlife crisis" in 1965 to refer to the phase of life when adults come face-to-face with their own mortality. "Crisis" speaks to how one responds to the fact that life is roughly half over. However, many experts don't believe that "crisis" is an appropriate term. More precisely, it marks a period of midlife *transitions*. People cope with these transitions in a variety of ways. Some take them in stride as a normal phase; others don't cope so well and may even slip into depression. The way a person reacts to middle age is strongly influenced by culture. Since the United States and other Western societies idolize youth, the thought of growing old often carries negative connotations. But in cultures that acknowledge "the splendor of old men is their gray head" (Prov. 20:29), advancing years bring esteem and rewards. In such places, midlife crisis is not nearly as evident—even nonexistent.

Some of the transitions typifying midlife include

- bodily changes associated with aging (including menopause);
- children leaving home (the "empty nest");
- the declining health or death of parents;
- milestone birthdays (those ending in zero or five); and
- birth of grandchildren

In addition to coping with these transitions, midlife also brings the tendency to look back on years past, reflecting on choices and opportunities—those taken and those missed. Problems arise when such thoughts bring a sense of disappointment, typically in areas related to

- career and employment;
- education;
- relationships, marriage, and family; and
- finances

Even a hint of regret, if left unchecked, can prove detrimental. And if we couple feelings of regret with the realization that we cannot recover time lost, we can find ourselves on a slippery slope leading to despair and desperation. In such circumstances, we can yearn to do something—*anything*—before it's too late. This can fuel anxious attempts to recover missed opportunities and reverse past choices as we scramble against our ever-present sense of working against the clock. When this happens we are inclined to make decisions in haste—some of which carry long-term consequences. This kind of response is never advantageous. Indeed, it can be destructive personally and to our loved ones. Our goal is peace, not panic. Ideally, we should glide into life's transitions in a positive, productive fashion. However, this requires coming to terms with three key issues: *loss, control,* and *hope.* Let's examine each by gaining insights from the life of the Old Testament prophet Daniel.

Loss

Experiencing loss is part of every phase of life. Yet aging brings with it more *occasions* to endure the experience. The way we respond to loss tends to change over time. In general, we become more poignant and reflective as we age, compared to our reactions as young adults or children. How, when, and where do we manifest loss? In all aspects of our being. Opportunities, relationships, and even time itself are fair game for its pain. The important thing is to process it in a healthy manner—irrespective of its source.

Those who are inclined to mourn the passing of time and opportunity can start reversing this outlook by considering how Daniel confronted reality: "Now from among those of the sons of Judah were Daniel, Hananiah, Mishael, and Azariah. To them the chief of the eunuchs gave names: he gave Daniel the name Belteshazzar; to Hananiah, Shadrach; to Mishael, Meshach; and to Azariah, Abed-Nego" (Dan. 1:6–7).

A mere teenager when Babylon conquered Daniel's homeland of Judah in 605 BC, Daniel remained there for the rest of his life. However, during the nation's seventy-year-long period of captivity, he never forgot his roots. Daniel fondly recalled the land of his people, particularly the temple in Jerusalem. Now from a natural standpoint, this was wartime, and "all is fair in love and war." The victors (Babylon) took the spoils of war, which included human capital like the bright young minds of Daniel and his friends. The Babylonians intended to brainwash them and indoctrinate them into their culture so these Jewish captives would willingly serve the empire. As Daniel 1:7 indicates, they even changed their Hebrew names. Yet their captivity involved more than the victor in war. At the forefront was a spiritual matter. This was God's judgment upon His covenant people who had rejected His precepts. Babylon was merely a tool for executing the verdict.

Yet while the Jewish *nation* was guilty, Daniel the *individual* was innocent. A righteous man, his devotion to God never wavered—even after Babylon took him captive, and even when such devotion placed his life in danger. So Daniel faced kidnapping, deportation, and a life sentence of serving in a pagan land, all for the crimes of others. If anyone could justify clinging to the pain of loss, it would have been Daniel. A delightful and prosperous life destined to be his—*if only!* So many possibilities. So many opportunities. All lost. Surely Daniel could have allowed this experience to lead him into the land of "if only." Once there, his *mind* would live in the same captivity as his *body*. However, as a man of wisdom, Daniel understood the futility of regret. Some losses can never be regained. We cannot change the past, nor what might have been and what can never be. Those who age gracefully understand and accept these truths.

Let's review some losses those in midlife and beyond often experience.

Lost opportunity

For some, adolescence is a difficult phase of life, a time when confusion and insecurity prevail. Even the most mild-mannered children can transform into rebels, and heretofore level-headed kids yield to negative peer pressure. Typically teens fail to comprehend much beyond the "here and now." The adolescent psyche fails to grasp the reality of projected outcomes, risk-to-benefit ratios, and long-term consequences. The young brain has not fully developed the capacity to factor such concepts into day-to-day decisions.

Unfortunately, during this tumultuous phase people can make choices that can impact the remainder of life. A case in point is cigarette smoking; most smokers initiate this habit before eighteen, usually at fourteen or fifteen. At that age people lack the insight to consider the consequences. Such questions as "What diseases might I develop if I start smoking?" and "How much money will this habit cost me?" don't cross the mind of a fourteen-year-old eager to impress his or her friends. In due season, when maturity reveals the folly of this decision, people must grapple with the monster of nicotine addiction (a battle best avoided!).

Adolescents also make crucial choices regarding education and careers. Some paid little attention to the advice of parents and school counselors or totally rejected it. Advice like "Stay in school," "Study hard," or "Think about your future" passed in one ear and out the other. Now, many of us know children born with "silver spoons" in their mouths (maybe you were one). They had parents with influence or affluence who could offset their foolishness. Such kids never worried about their grades or SAT scores suffering from too much partying. They didn't jeopardize their future, because Dad had power and influence, even over college admission boards. If your spoon happened to be stainless steel or plastic, you know choices made during the teen years could impact your entire future. One misguided decision might close a door of opportunity—and lock it forever.

However, even if you successfully negotiated the teen years and landed yourself a promising career, it is still common to look back and reflect on lost opportunities. Sometimes we selected a career because of the "extras," such as a nice benefits package or a generous pension. Or perhaps the location appealed to us, since settling there meant tasteful homes and superior schooling for the kids. Maybe you work for a family business, where you didn't choose your profession as much as inherited it. Many factors influence career choice, and many have nothing to do with enjoyment or passion. However, as the years go by, enjoyment and passion take on a greater degree of significance in life. This is when the seeds of regret bear the fruit of disillusionment and a desire for change.

For some, this need for change can instill a sense of urgency. Passing time means lost opportunities, a realization that can feel unsettling and provoke anxiety. How ought we to respond? Rationally, not radically. So if you're feeling "locked in" to a job or profession, before doing anything rash consider the following:

- Will a change affect my family? If your family depends on your income, then don't quit your job without having a plan to replace this financial support. If your family will need to forfeit a lifestyle they've grown accustomed to in order for you to achieve your goals, you should communicate this and elicit their agreement *before* implementing any changes.

- Is a change realistic? We are familiar with stories about the person who finally earns a college degree at eighty-five or ninety. Now, I'm all for achieving goals, and I applaud these seniors for their gump-tion. However, we will not see every dream we've ever dreamt manifested in our lifetime. It is up to us to use wisdom to discern between what is sensible and what is impractical. I have heard people use Paul's words from Philippians 4:13, "I can do all things through Christ who strengthens me," to validate self-centered or irrational decisions. So before taking Bible verses out of context, ask yourself: "Is this real-istic? Is it even feasible?"

- Are my emotions governing me? One of the nine fruits of the Holy Spirit listed in Galatians 5:22–23 is peace. One of God's Hebrew names is "Jehovah

Shalom," meaning the God of peace. When the Holy
Spirit governs us, peace prevails, even when our circumstances are not to our liking. Lost opportunities
can bring feelings of dissatisfaction, discontentment,
and disillusionment. Don't allow these emotions to
prevail! They will steal your peace and tempt you to
react in haste.

Certainly, we will face times of reflecting on missed opportunities. There is nothing wrong with that, provided we stay practical. For some, change is appropriate, even if it means returning
to school or relocating. At other times, change is unwise or simply
not possible. But rather than becoming frustrated by your status,
consider Daniel. He spent his entire working life in a strange land
and in a system that did not line up with his values. Surely he was
entitled to pine over lost opportunities. No one would blame him
for feeling frustrated, or "locked in" to a job that wasn't his heart's
desire. But as a man of great character, Daniel performed his work
with excellence. Recognize that all work is honorable. Replace discontentment with gratitude. Whatever your profession, do your
work with integrity and a spirit of peace.

Lost relationships

In his poem "When You Are Old," the legendary William B.
Yeats eloquently speaks to the matter of passing time and relationships that might have been:

> When you are old and grey and full of sleep,
> And nodding by the fire, take down this book,
> And slowly read, and dream of the soft look
> Your eyes had once, and of their shadows deep;
>
> How many loved your moments of glad grace,
> And loved your beauty with love false or true,

> But one man loved the pilgrim soul in you,
> And loved the sorrows of your changing face;
>
> And bending down beside the glowing bars,
> Murmur, a little sadly, how Love fled
> And paced upon the mountains overhead
> And hid his face amid a crowd of stars.[1]

Unlike other men, the writer didn't base his affection on the woman's outer beauty; looks are destined to fade with time. "Charm is deceitful and beauty is passing" is how Proverbs 31:30 confirms this truth (rather bluntly, in my opinion). Yet even though the object of his admiration didn't reciprocate Yeats's love, he responded with gentle and kind words instead of bitterness.

The sense of loss in relationships comes from many sources. Sometimes, as in the poem, there is a desire for a bond that never became a reality. Loss can be permanent—for instance, through death. Or it may come from a change in the *nature* of the relationship, as with divorce or the "empty nest" syndrome. Whatever the source, loss is inevitable. The take-home point from this poetry lesson is that we respond to loss with grace.

Death

Any loss is stressful. Even losing a job or "losing" your old neighborhood after relocating is emotionally draining. But the sense of loss that comes when a loved one dies can be devastating. Grief is a normal response. Contrary to what many believe, grief is *not* evidence of a weak faith. Naomi, David, and other heroes of the Bible all expressed sorrow in response to the death of a friend or family member. While everyone will not grieve in the same manner, there are typical stages of progression:

- *Denial.* Initially we may experience a period of detachment. Some describe it as feeling "numb," a time when they have yet to realize the full intensity of the loss.

An example would be a widow who plans her spouse's funeral in a calm, businesslike demeanor. She maintains her composure through the service, burial, and repast. The denial phase only ends when everything ends and she returns to a quiet home, all alone.

- *Bargaining.* The hallmark of bargaining is a rehashing of the "what ifs." Thoughts persist about all the variables that led to the outcome, and how they could have been changed. Even insignificant actions, either committed or omitted, become major points of reflection. Left unchecked, this stage leads to overwhelming feelings of guilt and regret.

- *Sadness.* In this phase, a person genuinely *feels* the void. There is nothing to deny, and no measure of bargaining will change things. Sadness prevails. Fatigue, insomnia, crying spells, anxiety, loss of appetite, and difficulty concentrating are all typical symptoms. They are also the early signs of depression, which can develop if this phase does not resolve itself within a reasonable period of time.

- *Anger.* This phase can be difficult to accept. Anger comes from feeling frustrated, helpless, and abandoned. The object of the anger, however, can be the deceased person, or even God Himself. Coming to terms with this phase requires a bit of soul-searching because it can bring on a sense of shame.

- *Acceptance.* This final phase is when grieving ends and healing begins. The person comes to terms with the loss and takes measures to adjust to the void. While never forgetting the loved one, the person is ready to embrace the future.

Keep in mind that these phases are *typical*, not *fixed* in stone. We make a big mistake when we try to standardize grief. Everyone responds in his or her own manner. We must be sensitive to this, especially in the things we say to console. Sometimes it's best to imitate Job's friends (that is, during the first week of their stay) and say nothing.

The goal is for grief to resolve itself over time. Some things will smooth the progression, while others delay it. When we deny our feelings rather than acknowledge them, we delay the process. Likewise, we can distract ourselves with work and other activities. It is fine to stay busy, but not if this busyness is a way to suppress emotions. Some people handle their pain by self-medicating with alcohol, drugs (including prescriptions) and even food. None of these approaches is beneficial. We facilitate healing by accepting the way we feel, however painful. Shedding tears is therapeutic, so don't suppress the urge to cry. Some people find journaling helpful. Of course, talking to a trusted friend or counselor is also a good idea.

While sadness is normal during the grieving process, sometimes the depressed mood does not resolve itself appropriately. This is when grieving leads to clinical depression. There is much overlap between what is normal and what is not, but in general the intensity and duration are important considerations. If the symptoms fail to subside over the course of months, then seek the advice of a health care professional. We revisit the topic of grief in greater detail in chapter 7.

Divorce

We can all agree on some aspects of divorce: it's not unusual, it can be messy, and disputes over money often cause it. But going beyond common knowledge to an objective analysis of the statistics is easier said than done. Many sources would have us believe the odds for a successful marriage are the same as a coin toss—50/50! It is no wonder many modern couples feel justified in skipping the altar altogether. Indeed, when it comes to divorce stats, some popular quotes are right on target:

- George Canning: "I can prove anything by statistics except the truth."

- Mark Twain: "Facts are stubborn, but statistics are more pliable."

- Vin Scully: "Statistics are used much like a drunk uses a lamppost: for support, not illumination."[2]

However, rather than deliberate on percentages and numbers, let's focus on relationship. Irrespective of the circumstances leading to the split, divorce represents loss. But unlike the loss that comes through death, where grief is the main response, divorce stirs up not only grief but more caustic emotions—bitterness, anger, a desire for vengeance, and jealousy once the ex finds someone new.

In his letter to the Ephesians, Paul said, "Let all bitterness, wrath, anger, clamor, and evil speaking be put away from you, with all malice" (Eph. 4:31). In particular, vengeance never belongs to us, but—according to Deuteronomy 32:35—is reserved for God. Whenever a relationship ends, all types of negative feelings will surface. But divorce in particular makes us susceptible to highly toxic emotions. Unlike severing ties with a business partner or even a friend, divorce represents a violation of a vow. The fact that a covenant has been broken serves to intensify the emotional impact.

No matter how painful the breakup, though, nobody wins when toxic emotions prevail. They especially affect children. An already challenging situation becomes even tougher for kids caught in the middle of a parental crossfire. It is not fair to try "winning" a child's support by berating the other parent. Whatever your feelings about your ex, she or he is still your child's mom or dad; for that reason alone respect is in order. Unfortunately, when people fail to process negative emotions, they trickle into subsequent relationships, setting the stage for more failure. This is why divorce rates for second and third marriages are higher than for first marriages. Toxic emotions can even destroy us physically and compromise our health. This is particularly true with respect to heart disease, something I discuss in detail in my book *Spiritual Secrets to a Healthy Heart*.

If you have experienced divorce, understand the importance of processing this loss. Even if you initiated the split and are relieved to be out of the relationship, it still represents a loss. The key to handling negative emotions is to recognize they have no authority over us—if love governs our hearts and actions. When we are quick to forgive, it prevents toxic emotions from gaining a stronghold in our lives. This may appear impossible, especially amid issues of betrayal or abuse, but never underestimate the power of grace. It gives us what we need to let go and move on.

The empty nest

My husband and I didn't have our first child until I was almost thirty. So while most of our friends are already "empty nesters," we still have a few years to go. Yet even as I wrote this chapter, we were in the midst of a poignant transition. Three of our four children were graduating—our oldest daughter from college, oldest son from high school, and youngest daughter from eighth grade. (Only child #3, our second-oldest son, skipped pomp and circumstance that year.) The eighth grade graduation was especially difficult. It was an emotional time because my husband and I had been actively involved with our daughter's elementary school for more than fifteen years. So this graduation marked the end of a significant phase of our lives. And while our connections to the faculty and other parents may not be permanently severed, they have certainly changed, and we feel the loss.

The empty nest syndrome is both a *real* transition where children physically leave the home as well as an *emotional* transition where parents come to terms with their departure. It can happen to any parent, although stay-at-home moms and dads are especially vulnerable. For some this period is a real struggle, but others live in joyful anticipation of the future. They feel no distress over an empty nest.

BIBLICAL INSIGHTS

> Now when Daniel knew that the writing was signed, he went home. And in his upper room, with his windows open toward Jerusalem, he knelt down on his knees three times that day, and prayed and gave thanks before his God, as was his custom since early days.
>
> —DANIEL 6:10

One thing Daniel's life demonstrates is how envy can be deadly. In this passage a jealous group of men finagled the passage of a law designed as Daniel's death sentence. Knowing of Daniel's righteousness, they persuaded the king to issue a decree making Daniel's kind of devotion a crime punishable by death. It required that "whoever petitions any god or man for thirty days, except you, O king, shall be cast into the den of lions" (Dan. 6:7). Bible students know the rest of the story: God prevents the lions from touching Daniel.

However, my point is not about God's power to deliver. I chose this verse because for me, the words paint a picture of solitude. Daniel went home—alone. Daniel got on his knees and prayed—alone. In fact, there is no record that Daniel had an immediate family. Scripture tells us that during captivity God not only permitted marriage; He encouraged it. God told Jeremiah the Israelites should build houses, get married, and have children—then make sure their kids did the same (see Jeremiah 29:4–6). Still, it appears Daniel had neither wife nor children. Which brings us to the subject of the empty nest. It is important to recognize that some people are like Daniel: they are empty nesters by default.

Of course, the reasons why people don't have children is as diverse as the individuals themselves. It ranges from personal choice to infertility, with a ton of factors in between. Whatever the circumstances, if you are childless, recognize that it is common to face emotional turmoil once middle age hits. You might find yourself struggling right along with the folks whose kids are leaving for college. And while there are a myriad of emotions, make a point to guard your heart against these three:

- Regret. It is easy to slip into the pit of regret and wallow there. The tragedy is that regret tarnishes our future by locking us into an unchangeable past. Don't allow it to get a stronghold.

- Envy. This one is deadly, as Daniel's story proves. To make matters worse, envy can be subtle and rationalized with ease. Check yourself and be brutally honest. If you find even an inkling of ill will toward people who have children, purge those toxic emotions right away.

- Unforgiveness. When infertility is the issue, forgive the people who ask foolish questions or make insensitive comments to you. When childlessness is because of a rash decision made in years past, forgive yourself for being shortsighted. And certainly if abortion is part of your testimony, cast that burden on the Lord because He loves you, and He cares. Whatever the source of pain, don't let bitterness take root. Forgive and move forward.

The empty nest brings with it an outpouring of feelings—some positive, others negative. This wide range of emotions surface because in addition to the youngest child's departure, other variables play a significant role. They include the following:

- The quality of the marriage. Some people handle problems by ignoring them, and marital problems are no exception. During child-rearing years, a house full of kids provides a convenient way to overlook the elephant in the room. Once the children leave, though, the status of the marriage—whether good or bad— surfaces. In some cases, there are identifiable problems within the relationship. In other cases, there's no specific offense, but in the quiet of a childless home an ominous sense of detachment surfaces. The fire is quenched and feelings toward the spouse shift into neutral, or are even bland. This happens because a couple took the time and attention needed to nurture the marriage and invested it in the children— year after year after year. Don't let this happen. Be proactive. Create a plan for how you will cultivate your relationship, beginning with the first positive pregnancy test! Remember, children should enhance the marriage, not destroy it.

- Single parenthood. In a healthy marriage, the husband and wife anticipate having more time and resources to invest in each other once their children leave. Loneliness is not a major problem, because spouses reallocate extra time toward each other. However, loneliness can pose a bigger issue for a single parent. In both cases the children will be missed, but their absence is not as painful when someone else is there to fill the void.

- Personal identity. If a parent's identity is "Kayla's Mom" or "Jordan's Dad," then what happens to the sense of self once the child becomes independent? The empty nest can expose a serious identity crisis where the parent struggles to find meaning and purpose. This problem is more common with stay-at-home parents.

- Guilt. All of our years pass swiftly, but particularly the parenting years. Because of this, the empty nest can be a time of intense remorse. Many parents feel guilty for not being more involved in their children's lives. Parents cannot recover time spent at the office or in other endeavors, and some deeply regret the lost opportunities.

- Life's stressors. The departure of children from the home often overlaps with other major life events, such as menopause, preparing for retirement, caring for aging parents, and dealing with the death of parents. These concurrent stressors will intensify the pain of the empty nest.

Whether through death, divorce, the empty nest, or other factors not listed here, relationships are destined to change over time. And change can usher in a host of emotions, such as grief, regret, anger, and despondency. We are often surrounded by constant reminders of past relationships, which can be good if it triggers positive reflections and warm memories. It is not so good when it stirs up negative emotions. Allow yourself time to process your feelings, especially grief and regret; they can be slow to resolve. Of course, you should deal immediately with anger, bitterness, and the desire for revenge. Purge yourself of these toxic emotions through the power of forgiveness. Finally, remember that loss can make one vulnerable to clinical depression. Be aware of the signs and symptoms, and don't be ashamed to seek advice from a health care professional.

Lost time

I doubt if Daniel kept a "bucket list," and even if he did, he wouldn't have called it that. Referring to a list of things a person would like to do before dying ("kicking the bucket"), the term became popular around 2006. The concept speaks to the matter of lost time. Each passing day means fewer opportunities for reaching dreams and fulfilling desires—whether it's travelling, skydiving, or learning a foreign language. The trend has become so popular that there are now websites and phone apps to help you create your own list.

I'm not too fond of the idea, even though I've done plenty of things that captured the essence of a bucket list. For instance, in 2014 I read Leo Tolstoy's *War and Peace*; my high school English teacher didn't include it on her list of required readings. Through the years it just became something I wanted to do—almost like a personal challenge. It took me six months to finish, but I did it, and I have no regrets.

What are my reservations about bucket lists? Problems arise when people draft a list in response to feelings of unrest or fear. Trust me when I tell you I would not have lost a minute of sleep had I never read *War and Peace*. Yes, it was something I wanted to do, but in the big scheme of things, it wasn't that important. I did not expect Tolstoy's words to bring my life to full circle, nor did they authenticate my existence. I didn't worry that it might be my "last chance" to read it. So for me, it was *nice* to do, but not *necessary*. And that's the key. If we make a list, it should simply be things we want to do if given the chance. Nothing frantic about it and no sense of urgency attached.

Since our days are finite, there is a limit to how much we can accomplish in a lifetime. Each day pulls us closer to the end and the time of no more opportunities. For some, this thought triggers anxiety. But those who have peace do not feel troubled or anxious. The real issue is not that we will miss the chance to do "fun stuff," but coming to terms with the cycle of life. If we haven't, then our list continually grows and becomes more outrageous.

Our task is to replace urgency with peace. Appreciate each day primarily for what it is and not for what you can accomplish. It's a day the Lord has made—so rejoice! Sure, keep a list of things you'd like to do, but don't let it govern you. More importantly, make a list of things you *will not* do—those habits, activities, and pervasive thoughts that are a genuine waste of time.

In addition, don't get caught up in all the things you want to do for *yourself.* Make a list of ways you can enrich the lives of others. These are just a few simple exercises to help replace anxiety with peace. Remember life still has meaning—even if you never climb the Himalayas.

CONTROL

Like high school and college students, medical students who have met graduation requirements can choose from several different courses during their last year. One of the clinical rotations I selected in my fourth year was geriatric medicine. At the time a rapidly growing specialty, I was seriously considering whether to select geriatrics as my field. The instructor was a spry Greek physician, older than most of his patients, a phenomenal teacher, and a delight to be around. At the end of the course, he traditionally treated his students to dinner at one of Chicago's finest Greek restaurants. (Needless to say, that pretty much sealed my decision to register.)

During that month I learned quite a bit about the physiology of aging. We also spent a great deal of time delving into the psychosocial aspects of growing old—for me, the best part of the course. One point our professor emphasized was the issue of control and how forfeiting control is a fundamental part of the aging process. Even though inevitable, it is nevertheless difficult to accept.

BIBLICAL INSIGHTS

So they answered and said before the king, "That Daniel, who is one of the captives from Judah, does not show due regard for you, O king, or for the decree that you have signed, but makes his petition three times a day."

—DANIEL 6:13

Involuntarily shunted off to a foreign land, Daniel experienced insult on top of injury. In addition to captivity, his permanent injury meant remaining in Babylon for his entire life. The insult: his captors wanted total control of every aspect of his existence. Things that were entirely personal, and matters that bore no impact on his ability to serve the Babylonian government, came under attack. His captors did not honor his God and wanted to wipe out his allegiance.

In the passage I quoted earlier from chapter 1, they gave Daniel food that did not line up with God's law. In that instance, Daniel negotiated a peaceful resolution that permitted him to eat foods that were acceptable. Years later, Daniel's prayer life came under attack. The verse I just quoted reveals the plan to destroy him. Certainly, those behind the scheme were motivated more by jealousy and hatred than a desire to control the way he worshipped. Irrespective of their motives, however, the end result landed Daniel in a situation beyond his control. If he had his "druthers" he would not have chosen an overnight stay in a lion's den! Yet despite this, he trusted a God with full dominion. The next morning the authorities found him very much alive, in the presence of some very hungry lions! We learn from Daniel to trust God in *all* circumstances—whether we're in full control or completely powerless. Rest in the knowledge that God sees us, loves us, and is faithful.

When we consider issues of control, sometimes we need to laugh to keep from crying. The similarities between infancy and old age yield a prime example. In the story of Oedipus, the mythological sphinx presents a riddle that speaks to this full circle: "What walks on four feet in the morning, two feet in the afternoon, and three feet at night?" In the story, many met their death by failing to solve the riddle, but Oedipus knew the answer: man. In infancy we crawl on all fours, in adulthood we walk on two legs, and in old age, we use a cane. Both the baby and the senior are prone to an unsteady gait and need assistance to walk. Here are a few other parallels (remember—laugh, don't cry!):

- *Bladder control.* Potty training is a milestone everyone appreciates, since it can take a few years before parents are finally diaper free. But once those parents become grandparents, the diapers return. And they aren't just for grandbaby, but for Grandma and Grandpa too!

- *Sleep.* "Oh look, he's fallen asleep." The "he" of that endearing comment might be young or old. Nodding off at any given moment—even inopportune moments—is a common feature of both.

- *Daycare centers.* Parent send young children to daycare against their cries of protest: "Why can't I stay home!" Children send elderly parents to daycare against their cries of protest: "Why can't I stay home!"

These all speak, in a bittersweet sort of way, to the loss of control that accompanies aging. It is manifested in so many aspects of life, from interpersonal relationships to health to everything in between. We lose control of authority over our children when they become adults. If our cognitive function declines, we lose the ability to live independently and manage our own affairs. While there are ways to intervene, we cannot fully control bodily changes such as skin texture, hair loss, and fat replacing muscle. One of the most difficult aspects comes with chronic disease where we, in essence, relinquish control of our health.

Throughout the life span, things happen against our will, meaning we are subjected to circumstances we are powerless to control. With age, the list grows and the frequency increases. Certainly, "Type A" personalities will struggle in this area more than those who are easygoing. The challenge is to guard your heart against frustration, which will ultimately lead to bitterness. Make a decision to respond like Daniel. Accept those things you cannot change, go with the flow, and trust God.

HOPE

Since there is always a bigger picture, hope keeps our focus on it. Being hopeful is not a feeling but a decision of the will. It is not an emotional experience but an attitude we choose to maintain. It motivates us to stay on track, maintain a positive outlook, and start each day with grace. One reason I selected Psalm 8:4 to open this chapter is because it is a wonderful reminder of our reason for hope. The awesome Creator of the universe is "mindful" of us! He has given us hope for the present, and then secured our hope for eternity through Jesus Christ.

BIBLICAL INSIGHTS

> I was watching in the night visions, and behold, One like the Son of Man, coming with the clouds of heaven! He came to the Ancient of Days, and they brought Him near before Him. Then to Him was given dominion and glory and a kingdom, that all peoples, nations, and languages should serve Him. His dominion is an everlasting dominion, which shall not pass away, and His kingdom the one which shall not be destroyed.
> —DANIEL 7:13–14

Daniel recognized there was more to the equation of life than "me + my circumstances." How can I be so sure? Because throughout his long life, there is no evidence that Daniel grew discouraged, or that his commitment to God ever waned. He maintained hope. To be sure, many would describe his situation as hopeless—a lifetime sentence despite his innocence represents a valid reason for despondency. But Daniel didn't become disheartened since he knew his *purpose* was larger than his *person*. Unlike the prophet

Jonah, Daniel wasn't self-centered, the key to maintaining hope. We must understand the big picture is all that really matters, and its focal point is not self. Daniel describes this big picture in chapters 7–12, the visionary portion of his book. God is the big picture. The reason for hope appears in verse 7:13: He is sovereign, and His kingdom is eternal!

In the Book of Lamentations, Jeremiah writes of God's compassion and love. These are renewed every morning because He is faithful (see Lamentations 3:23). Irrespective of our age, He is faithful. Regardless of our station in life, He is faithful. God's promises don't lose their validity over the course of a life span. They are unfailing when we are young and when we're old. However, while each day holds new promises and possibilities, the aging process can blind some people to this truth. Instead of embracing a new day with hope, they develop a sense of futility, cynicism, and pessimism.

One way to rejuvenate hope is through investing in people. Sow seeds in the future. Leave a legacy. Interestingly, the natural laws of sowing and reaping teach a great lesson about hope. We prepare the soil and cast our seeds before seeing a harvest. We plant because we have faith in God's laws of sowing and reaping. If we do our part and plant seeds, harvest time strengthens our hope. Remember what takes place in the natural world is reflected in our spiritual lives. Sow seeds of blessings in future generations. Share your wisdom and knowledge, invest your time and resources, and look for opportunities to bless someone else. By doing so, you will surely reap a harvest of hope.

Chapter 7

MENTAL HEALTH PART 1: DEPRESSION AND ANXIETY

The LORD knows the thoughts of man...

—PSALM 94:11

ASK THE AVERAGE person, "What's your major fear about getting older?," and there is a good chance their answer will have something to do with the mind. Memory loss, confusion, mental illness, and losing the capacity to manage personal affairs are high on the list of most people's concerns. Many are not as worried about a decline in *physical* health as they are about maintaining *mental* capacity. Just watch the countenance of anyone giving a status report on an elderly relative. If he or she is still alert and mentally capable, a smile appears as the person proclaims: "They're sharp as a tack." Of course, the ability to live independently and "still get around" requires physical *and* cognitive function. Yet we tend to be more impressed with the latter, which I will address more fully in chapter 8.

Declining mental health is more than a personal fear. It creates challenges on all fronts, especially for family members. Cognitive or psychiatric impairment intensifies the burden on caregivers. The risk of harm and life-threatening injury skyrockets in the face of memory loss, dementia, or mental illness. Reports of house fires ignited by stovetops left unattended, water damage from faucets left turned on, and death from exposure after getting lost in bad weather are common.

163

In this chapter and the next, we will examine matters relating to the brain and the mind. We'll start with the two most common mental health disorders seen in the general population: depression and anxiety. These conditions are not age specific but are seen in children and young adults as well. Then we will look at the areas of memory loss and dementia, problems which definitely become more prevalent with the passing years.

MENTAL HEALTH

Depression

Depression is common among Americans. In the 2008 National Health and Nutrition Examination Survey, nearly 7 percent of participating adults reported moderate to severe symptoms of depression during the two weeks prior to taking the survey. By 2030, it is projected to be the leading cause of disability in developed countries, even surpassing the burdens caused by physical conditions. Although the average age of onset is the early thirties, it is often diagnosed during the teen years. It is not a disease of older people per se. However, aging will definitely increase the odds of developing it. This is because chronic medical illnesses (i.e., diabetes, heart disease, and cancer) and such traumatic life events as the death of a loved one are independent risk factors for depression. Both happen more often among older people.

There are also racial differences. Compared with other races, African Americans are less likely to develop depression, but when it occurs it tends to be more chronic and debilitating. With respect to gender, new data has emerged that challenges the idea that depression is predominantly a woman's disease. Much like heart disease, it turns out the signs and symptoms of depression differ between the sexes. Common manifestations of depression in men are anger, aggression, substance abuse, and risk-taking behavior. However, tools that screen for depression traditionally use such factors as sadness, a change in appetite, and insomnia; while common in depressed women, they might not be a problem for depressed men. This could explain why, using the current diagnostic criteria, women are twice as likely to be diagnosed with depression.

Although depression is extremely common, far too many people remain "silent sufferers." They dismiss the symptoms, don't seek help, or refuse treatment. Why? One reason is a general lack of knowledge about mental health, particularly mood disorders like major depression, dysthymia, and bipolar disorder. I find this is especially the case among older adults. Younger adults have apparently benefitted from recent popular campaigns aimed at increasing mental health awareness.

A common misconception is that our mood is entirely voluntary and under our complete control. A second misconception is that a person's mood should parallel his or her life's circumstances. Sometimes beliefs have an inkling of truth but are not entirely accurate, which is certainly the case here. Yes, to a large extent we have the capacity to govern the way we feel. This explains why behavioral therapy works so well as a means of treating depression. But mood disorders result from chemical imbalances in the brain. We can't voluntarily regulate the concentration of substances like serotonin, dopamine, and norepinephrine in the same way we voluntarily control the movement of our arms and legs. Because we are in command of our muscles, when we want to move, we move. Mental health disorders are different. A person may *want* to feel good but they *don't*—and it's not their fault.

The other misconception is that mood should reflect circumstances. Many believe how we *feel* ought to line up with how it *is*— if things are going badly, the mood should be bad; if things are going good, the mood should be good. This again has a hint of truth. Adjustment Disorder with Depressed Mood, for instance, is diagnosed in the context of a stressful event like the death of a loved one. In this case, time and an adequate support system can resolve the problem; medications and psychotherapy are not required. But it is a mistake to believe that mood disorders only occur in the face of hardship. Again, they are the result of chemical imbalances, which can happen to anyone, even to people with pleasant, stress-free lives.

Then there's the issue of stigma. In my practice, I find this is far more problematic with older adults than younger men and women. And it is a serious problem! There have been times when I have convinced a patient that depression is a *medical* problem, not a character flaw. But social stigma still poses a barrier to treatment.

Take the woman in her early sixties I cared for several years ago. She suffered from major depression but refused to take antidepressants. By any standard, her life was good: she was in decent health, financially secure, and had a great husband, kids, and grandkids. Her "ideal" life made her even more ashamed of her feelings. So I spent quite a bit of time dispelling the notion fixed in her mind: "What do I have to be depressed about?"

Finally she agreed to take medication, which felt like a major breakthrough in her understanding of the disease. However, on a subsequent visit, I discovered the stigma remained. Yes, she was taking the antidepressant and felt much better. Her only complaint was how inconvenient it was to get the prescription filled. I didn't understand why that would present a problem. After much coaxing, she confessed. A customer at the same drug store for many years, she had developed a friendly relationship with the pharmacist. Although he processed all her "regular" medicines, she didn't give him the prescription for the antidepressant. Instead, she drove to a pharmacy in neighboring Indiana to get it filled. Her embarrassment over her depression was so immense that she desperately wanted to maintain anonymity.

I was glad she was taking medication, despite the unnecessary mileage. But it troubled me that such stigma and shame persist, even in the twenty-first century. This ought not be! If by chance you could imagine yourself doing something as radical as my patient, consider the following:

- A diagnosis of depression does not reflect a person's character any more than a diagnosis of arthritis or hypertension.

- There is a strong genetic predisposition. Some people are prone to depression because it's embedded in their DNA.

- Many celebrities have depression. Some famous actors, musicians, politicians, and athletes have written books sharing their struggles.

- Ignoring depression can adversely affect your livelihood. It is common for people to lose their jobs because of reduced productivity and absenteeism—expected outcomes when sufferers dismiss their depression.

- Treating depression will improve your overall health. Diabetes, asthma, heart disease, and most other medical conditions are negatively affected by mental health disorders.

- Treating depression will improve your relationships. This disease makes it difficult (if not impossible) to be the best friend, coworker, parent, or spouse you can possibly be.

- Remember you're not alone. Most people with depression have some degree of embarrassment about their diagnosis. But since it's so common, it's quite possible the very people you wouldn't want to know have struggled with it themselves!

The combination of ignorance and stigma poses a serious barrier to the diagnosis and treatment of *any* mental health disorder, including major depression. But unfortunately, the patient is not the only reason why depression goes overlooked. Sometimes (actually, quite often) the health care provider is the one who drops the ball. In fact, physicians who are not psychiatrists may miss the diagnosis in more than half the people who visit their offices with signs and symptoms of depression.

This is partially explained by the fact that depression's *physical* manifestations (for example, fatigue and body aches) may be the main complaint. If the health care provider is not astute (or if he or she is rushed, which is a separate issue), then he or she might fail to connect the dots tying vague physical symptoms to a mental health disorder. Because of this the US Preventive Services Task Force now recommends screening adults for depression, provided a comprehensive care team is in place to provide treatment and follow-up care.

BIBLICAL INSIGHTS

> I am the man who has seen affliction by the rod of His wrath. He has led me and made me walk in darkness and not in light. Surely He has turned His hand against me time and time again throughout the day. He has aged my flesh and my skin, and broken my bones. He has besieged me and surrounded me with bitterness and woe. He has set me in dark places like the dead of long ago.
>
> —LAMENTATIONS 3:1–6

Jeremiah served as a priest and prophet during a tragic period in Judah's history. After years of idolatry and rebellion, the Lord judged the nation and used Babylon to administer the sentence and take the Israelites captive. Jeremiah grieved over the condition of his people, a calamity that could have been entirely prevented had they heeded the call to repent. However, Jeremiah cried for another reason: his kinsmen punished him for speaking the truth. It is fitting, then, that Jeremiah is known as the "weeping prophet" and his second book is called "Lamentations."

In the above passage, Jeremiah gives a vivid description of his experience. His words suggest he has a

legitimate complaint against God. Though not personally guilty of any idolatry or rebellion, nevertheless he
notes the following:

- God is angry with me.
- God has placed me in darkness.
- God is acting like my enemy.
- I am physically affected by the way God
  has dealt with me (such as premature aging
  and body aches).
- I feel anger and sadness as a result of His
  actions.

Jeremiah brings to light how he feels and how
he has processed the events of his life. Based on his
words, one might be tempted to diagnose him with
major depression. I don't agree. Keep in mind that a
depressing situation is not the same as major depression. Difficult times can certainly make us vulnerable
to mood disorders, but it is not a cause-and-effect relationship. Plenty of people with major depression lead
lives of minimal stress, ones some would consider ideal.

While Jeremiah describes his pain sincerely, his
authenticity does not mean he misunderstood God's
purpose. He knew God's chastisement reflected His
love. God punished with a *rod* to correct, not a *sword* to
sever ties. His purpose was not to abandon the children
of Israel but to lead them in the right direction. And
though painful, the means of correction would prove
beneficial in the long run. Through it all, they were still
the apple of His eye. Proof that Jeremiah understood
this appears a few verses later: "Through the LORD's
mercies we are not consumed, because His compas-
sions fail not. They are new every morning; great is
Your faithfulness. 'The LORD is my portion,' says my
soul, 'therefore I hope in Him!'" (Lam. 3:22–24).

When tragedy strikes, some will blame God—
even reject Him. Not so with Jeremiah. Yes, he was

anguished, but because he embraced God's *purpose* for his pain, he endured it with a sound mind. Sometimes, though adversity and calamity are the order of the day, draw encouragement from them. Learn and grow from every experience. Understand that in all times and in all circumstances, God is faithful!

SCREENING FOR DEPRESSION

There are several screening tools for major depression. The Patient Health Questionnaire–2 (PHQ–2) consists of only two questions, which call for a yes or no response. It takes less than a minute to complete and is appropriate for all adults, with or without symptoms. The first question addresses mood. The second question relates to the symptom of "anhedonia," which happens when someone stops engaging in enjoyable activities *for no apparent reason.* In other words, it isn't because of such factors as a lack of money or lack of time; they just don't feel like having fun anymore. Anhedonia is a definite red flag for depression. The PHQ–2 asks:

- Over the past two weeks, have you felt down, depressed, hopeless?

- Over the past two weeks, have you felt little interest or pleasure in doing things?

If the answer to both questions is no, depression is so unlikely no further screening is necessary. But a yes response to one or both is considered a positive screen—highly sensitive for major depression. In this instance, delving into more details is helpful. The SALSA questions are a useful next step because they focus on the common symptoms of depression:

S: Sleep disturbances

A: Anhedonia

L, S: Low Self-esteem

A: Appetite changes

A positive response to at least two of the four SALSA questions essentially confirms depression.[1] If either the PHQ–2 or the SALSA is positive, it calls for a complete diagnostic assessment.

The PHQ–2 and SALSA are appropriate for adults of all ages. Some tools, however, are specifically designed for the geriatric population. As mentioned, depression is more commonly seen among younger adults, but seniors are at high risk in the presence of concurrent problems such as chronic medical illnesses, loss of cognitive function, or a decline in vision or hearing. Additionally, residents in assisted living or skilled nursing facilities have a heightened risk for depression. When this is the case, a screening tool like the Geriatric Depression Scale is appropriate. The long version of this scale is comprised of thirty questions; the short form reproduced below has only half that number.

Choose the best answer for how you have felt over the past week:

1. Are you basically satisfied with your life? YES / **NO**

2. Have you dropped many of your activities and interests? **YES** / NO

3. Do you feel that your life is empty? **YES** / NO

4. Do you often get bored? **YES** / NO

5. Are you in good spirits most of the time? YES / **NO**

6. Are you afraid that something bad is going to happen to you? **YES** / NO

7. Do you feel happy most of the time? YES / **NO**

8. Do you often feel helpless? **YES** / NO

9. Do you prefer to stay at home, rather than going out and doing new things? **YES** / NO

10. Do you feel you have more problems with memory than most? **YES** / NO

11. Do you think it is wonderful to be alive now? YES / **NO**

12. Do you feel pretty worthless the way you are now? **YES** / NO

13. Do you feel full of energy? YES / **NO**

14. Do you feel that your situation is hopeless? **YES** / NO

15. Do you think that most people are better off than you are? **YES** / NO

BOLD responses indicate a problem. A score of five or more is highly suggestive of depression and should be followed with a more detailed interview. A score of ten or more essentially seals the diagnosis.[2]

TREATING DEPRESSION

The approach to treating depression depends on several variables, including the severity of the symptoms, personal preference, and the level of functional impairment. The latter refers to such things as maintaining productivity at work, getting things done around the house, and engaging with family and friends. Barring the need for inpatient care, or an emergent intervention because of severe symptoms or suicidal thoughts, the average person with depression can be managed by his or her primary care provider. There are four approaches to treatment:

- Self-management (minimal symptoms)
- Psychotherapy (mild symptoms)

- Medications (moderate to severe symptoms)

- Psychotherapy and medications combined (severe symptoms)

SELF-MANAGEMENT

For nearly every medical condition—whether affecting physical health or mental health—optimal care includes a component of self-management. I like to think of self-management as "empowerment care." It poses the challenge, "What can I do *for* myself, to *help* myself?" Anyone with major depression, no matter the severity, should be encouraged to engage in self-management. With self-management for problems like diabetes and heart disease, such steps as a healthy diet, adequate exercise, and smoking cessation come to mind. All of these—especially exercise—play a role in mental health.

The basis for self-management is education. As mentioned, in the mental health arena a lack of understanding and stigmatization represent huge challenges. There are many resources available, ranging from written materials to online information to support groups. For mild depression, tapping into such resources often provides sufficient therapy.

Self-management includes such steps as reserving time throughout the day—even if only a few minutes—to relax and unwind, and making specific plans for enjoyable activities. Learning to divide large problems into smaller components helps too. It guards against feeling overwhelmed and helpless, which can adversely affect the mood. Since depression plays a role in self-esteem, it is a good idea to make positive affirmations to counter negative thoughts. Memorizing Bible verses is especially beneficial. Look in the mirror and remind yourself of who you are in God's sight. Go ahead: recite His promises out loud!

Finally self-management for major depression includes physical activity. A good workout benefits the entire body and is a necessary component of total wellness. Along with time set aside for exercise, it is vital to increase the amount of physical activity in daily activities. For example, take the stairs instead of the elevator, walk somewhere, or ride a bike instead of driving. Physical activity is discussed in greater detail in chapters 3 and 9.

PSYCHOTHERAPY

In cases of mild to moderate depression, self-management with structured psychotherapy is the first line of treatment. Traditional psychotherapy is provided by a trained therapist or psychologist to individuals, or within a group setting. Typically a person receives about a dozen one-hour sessions over the course of three to six months. However, technology has broadened the options. Now, computer-based psychotherapy is available and is considered as beneficial as a face-to-face encounter.

The following are types of psychotherapy with proven efficacy:

- *Behavioral activation:* this form encourages a person to increase the amount of time spent thinking about and engaging in enjoyable activities.

- *Cognitive therapy:* one objective of this form is to change the manner of thinking, specifically with regard to thoughts that are pessimistic or self-critical.

- *Cognitive-behavioral therapy:* this is the most common form, incorporating positive thoughts with pleasurable activities.

- *Problem-solving therapy:* this helps people to manage seemingly insurmountable challenges by breaking them into smaller, more easily solvable problems.

- *Interpersonal therapy:* this type focuses on interpersonal conflicts and ways to resolve them.

Keep in mind, psychotherapy is a structured discipline administered by trained professionals. Although family members and friends may offer good advice, their interventions are not the same as psychotherapy. Likewise, counseling provided by a pastor or church leader—unless the person is licensed in this area—does not constitute psychotherapy. Yes, such support is beneficial, but it should never replace professional help. Improvement should be evident in two months, and remission within four months. If this does not take place, medications should be added.

MEDICATIONS

Several medications are available for treating moderate to severe depression. These can be used alone, or in combination with psychotherapy. In years past a psychiatrist usually prescribed such medications, but this is not the case anymore. Today general medical physicians and other primary care providers write about 75 percent of antidepressant prescriptions.

The main categories of prescription antidepressants are as follows:

- Selective Serotonin Reuptake Inhibitors (SSRIs): citalopram (Celexa), escitalopram (Lexapro), fluoxetine (Prozac), paroxetine (Paxil), sertraline (Zoloft)

- Serotonin-Norepinephrine Reuptake Inhibitors (SNRIs): venlafaxine (Effexor), desvenlafaxine (Pristiq), duloxetine (Cymbalta), levomilnacipran (Fetzima)

- Tricyclic Antidepressants: amitriptyline, desipramine (Norpramin), doxepin (Silenor), imipramine (Tofranil), nortriptyline (Pamelor), protriptyline (Vivactil), trimipramine (Surmontil)

- Monoamine Oxidase Inhibitors: isocarboxazid (Marplan), phenelzine (Nardil), selegiline (Emsam), tranylcypromine (Parnate)

- Others: amoxapine, bupropion (Wellbutrin), maprotiline, mirtazapine (Remeron), nefazodone, trazodone (Oleptro), vilazodone (Viibryd), vortioxetine (Brintellix)

The choice of therapy is based on several factors, including side effects, personal preference, and the potential for drug interactions with other prescriptions. SSRIs are usually the medication of first choice. Keep in mind that antidepressant medications don't have an immediate effect! It may take as long as two months to notice any difference, so it is important to continue taking them, even with no apparent initial response. Only about half of people treated with antidepressants respond to the first medication prescribed. If there is no improvement in three months, try a different medication.

Alternative and complementary therapies for depression include St. John's wort and light therapy. St. John's wort is not FDA approved but may be similarly effective with fewer side effects than standard medications. It does, however, interact with several prescription medications, and some of these reactions can be quite serious. Check with your primary health care provider to make sure it is safe to take. Bright light therapy can be beneficial, especially during the winter months when hours of daylight are reduced, particularly for those in northern climates.

The final factor on depression is bereavement. Growing older opens the door to many experiences, both positive and negative. It certainly brings plenty of opportunities to grieve, since the number of funerals attended reflects age. This includes the loss of close friends and family members; 30 percent of men and women over age sixty-five have experienced the death of a spouse.

In recent years, considerable discussion has revolved around clarifying what constitutes a "normal" grief response. Surely it is appropriate to feel sad after the loss of a loved one. But for some people, irrespective of age, intense sadness and other troubling symptoms persist for an unusually long period. They find themselves "locked" into the tragedy and unable to move forward with life. When this happens, normal bereavement slips into what is called complicated grief, where there is a persistent yearning for the deceased, or even a denial of their death. People with complicated grief may have stable periods interspersed with times of heightened distress—particularly around holidays, birthdays, and anniversaries. While the prevalence is not firmly established, it is estimated to affect about 4 percent of the general population, and nearly 7 percent of seniors.

BIBLICAL INSIGHTS

> Also the word of the LORD came to me, saying, "Son of man, behold, I take away from you the desire of your eyes with one stroke; yet you shall neither mourn nor weep, nor shall your tears run down. Sigh in silence, make no mourning for the dead; bind your turban on your head, and put your sandals on your feet; do not cover your lips, and do not eat men's bread of sorrow." So I spoke to the people in the morning, and at evening my wife died; and the next morning I did as I was commanded. And the people said to me, "Will you not tell us what these things signify to us, that you behave so?"
> —EZEKIEL 24:15–19

One characteristic of the Old Testament prophets (except for Jonah) was their willingness to accept that their mission ranked as more important than their lives. God's plan represented their number-one priority, even when God asked them to carry out unusual, sometimes embarrassing assignments. Take Isaiah, who walked naked and barefoot for three years to symbolize the coming shame of Egypt and Ethiopia (see Isaiah 20:3–4). The Lord told Hosea to marry the unfaithful harlot named Gomer (see Hosea 1:2). Hosea endured shame and humiliation to demonstrate to the people how much God loved them in spite of their idolatry. And the passage from Ezekiel reveals the prophet's calling to fulfill an especially painful task that would paint a picture of

God's message—He took the life of Ezekiel's wife and then forbade him to grieve.

Ezekiel accomplished this task. The people were intrigued by his behavior, and their fascination set the stage for a prophetic message to go forth. However, my goal is not to give examples of unwavering obedience—though that is indeed the case. It is not to show how God used a variety of methods to get his point across—although that is also the case. My point is this: there is nothing wrong with showing grief when a loved one dies. It's *normal*. Ezekiel drew attention to himself because his behavior was *abnormal*. He *didn't* express sadness, when sadness was the appropriate response.

Remember God's assignment to Ezekiel was a real "mission impossible." God called the prophet to suppress his pain and behave in an unexpected manner. But the call to Ezekiel does not apply to us. We know from this passage and others that grief is a normal response to loss. When confronted with the death of a loved one, allow yourself to grieve. When friends and family members lose a loved one, allow them to grieve. Sometimes as believers we assume our hope for the *future* ought to instantly alleviate any pain in the *present*. Yet even with an eternal hope, our hearts are subject to sorrow. Keep in mind that Ezekiel's task was uniquely his. Thankfully, God allows us to mourn.

The clinical arena features a long, challenging history of defining what constitutes normal vs. abnormal grieving. But in an honorable attempt to prevent bereavement from being classified as a mental health disorder, many people with an *abnormal* response have been overlooked. For this reason, in the fifth and most recent edition of the *Diagnostic and Statistical Manual of Mental Disorders (DSM-5)*, the American Psychiatric Association addresses complicated grieving by including Persistent Complex Bereavement Disorder as a condition warranting attention.

In normal grieving, sorrow tends to abate after six to eight months. But in the setting of complicated grief, distress and impairment persists. Researchers have identified six symptoms that give clues that grieving is not progressing normally:

- A yearning for and a preoccupation with thoughts of the deceased

- Feeling angry and bitter

- Feelings of shock and disbelief

- Becoming estranged from others

- Hallucinations of the deceased

- Behavioral changes (e.g., avoiding things that are reminders of the deceased, or seeking to be in close proximity to them)[3]

Strong social ties to friends and family help ensure that bereavement progresses normally. However, several circumstances increase the chance of complicated grief. Men and women who already have a mental health disorder like depression are at high risk. The conditions surrounding the death play a role, particularly if the person was absent during the days preceding death. The nature of the relationship is a contributing factor. Guilt, unresolved conflict, and a "love-hate" type of bond all predispose a person to complicated grief.

Men and women who served as the primary caregiver of the deceased are at especially high risk. When the physical and emotional toll of caring for a sick spouse or relative comes to an end, death stirs up a host of conflicting emotions. The caregiver often has a strong sense of relief because the nonstop burden lifts. At the same time, there can be intense guilt over having those feelings of relief. It's as if feeling good, fresh, and unburdened are in some way disrespectful to the dead person's memory.

Finally, no matter what the circumstances, the death of a loved one can prove draining physically, mentally, and emotionally. And there is no "quick fix" to the pain that accompanies loss. Yes, it will diminish over time, but there is no way to speed up the process. Patience, endurance, and strong social support are generally sufficient, but not for everyone. It's important to be aware of the signs that healing may not be progressing normally, and then seek help.

Anxiety

More than thirty million Americans have faced an anxiety disorder at some point in their lifetimes. But even though anxiety and depression are the two most common mental health disorders, they often go undetected. In recent years, various campaigns have helped to draw attention to both conditions. However, with respect to public awareness, anxiety disorder lags far behind depression.

Like depression, anxiety is not age specific. While diagnosed more frequently in younger adults, the age discrepancy is not entirely accurate. The problem is often overlooked in older adults. Anxiety disorders are twice as prevalent as dementia, and at least four times more prevalent than major depression. In older adults, risk factors include female gender, singleness, lower education, and the presence of three or more chronic medical illnesses.

Several conditions fall under the umbrella of anxiety disorders:

- General Anxiety Disorder (GAD). This is the most common type. People with GAD are tense, uneasy, and worry excessively, even when there is little cause for concern.

- Social Anxiety Disorder. People with social anxiety have extreme self-consciousness and distress in public or at social gatherings.

- Post-traumatic Stress Disorder (PTSD). PTSD causes long-lasting and typically frightening thoughts of a past traumatic event.

- Panic Disorder. The sudden onset of terror and feelings of impending doom are typical features. Physical symptoms include chest pain, palpitations, a sensation of choking, and shortness of breath.

- Obsessive Compulsive Disorder (OCD). People with OCD have constant fearful thoughts that compel them to perform rituals or routines. An example is excessive hand washing because of a fear of germs.

Compared to adolescents and younger adults, older adults are more likely to complain of the *physical* manifestations of anxiety than its effect on feelings and emotions. This makes sealing the diagnosis a challenge, especially in the face of concurrent medical problems. For instance, if a patient comes to my office complaining of chest pain, it draws my attention to the heart, especially if the individual is at risk for cardiovascular disease. Likewise, if the person is experiencing shortness of breath, I will focus on the lungs or other *medical* causes. Even though anxiety disorder could be the culprit, I am still likely to order tests to rule out a medical condition. Depending on the circumstances, I might even admit the patient to the hospital. Granted, there is nothing wrong with being cautious. But this explains why mental health disorders can prove elusive in older adults. It also explains why annual health care costs related to late-life anxiety are so high, exceeding $42 billion.

Anxiety disorders have a peak onset between ages eighteen and forty. When they develop later in life, 90 percent of the time they will manifest as either general anxiety disorder or social anxiety disorder. When illness, frailty, and loss coincide with the aging process, it sets the stage for a mind-set of vulnerability—even fear. These kinds of feelings can trigger anxiety. People who have little social support and people with other medical or psychiatric illnesses are especially susceptible.

The main symptom of general anxiety disorder is worry. Of

course, some situations can cause even folks with extreme confidence to lose a little sleep. We're all prone to feeling waves of apprehension occasionally. But GAD is different—more intense, even disabling. Some of the hallmarks include the following:

- Symptoms last over six months
- Worry extends into several different areas (e.g., finances, health, relationships)
- The person is not able to stop worrying
- It includes physical symptoms (e.g., fatigue, headache, muscle tension, insomnia, restlessness)
- The worrying interferes with normal functions (e.g., job performance, socializing, handling personal affairs)

Likewise, social anxiety disorder is more than just shyness. It features excessive self-consciousness while in public and a fear of being judged negatively. Not surprisingly, adults with social anxiety tend to isolate themselves to minimize the symptoms.

BIBLICAL INSIGHTS

Now it happened as they went that He entered a certain village; and a certain woman named Martha welcomed Him into her house. And she had a sister called Mary, who also sat at Jesus' feet and heard His word. But Martha was distracted with much serving, and she approached Him and said, "Lord, do You not care that my sister has left me to serve alone? Therefore tell her to help me." And Jesus answered and said to her, "Martha, Martha, you are worried and troubled about many things. But one thing is needed, and Mary has chosen that good part, which will not be taken away from her."

—LUKE 10:38–42

I am sure I'm not alone here. Have you ever heard a sermon, nodded in agreement, and maybe even thanked the preacher for the timely message—only to stumble in the same area before next Sunday? It looks like that's what happened to Martha. She and her siblings were good friends with Jesus. They respected Him, held His ministry in high regard, and often welcomed Him as a guest. So it is quite likely that Martha heard Jesus deliver the Sermon on the Mount. Even if she wasn't there, though, it is safe to assume she knew its key points—including the issue of worry. In that sermon, Jesus said, "Therefore do not worry, saying, 'What shall we eat?' or 'What shall we drink?' or 'What shall we wear?'...But seek first the kingdom of God and His righteousness, and all these things shall be added to you." (Matt. 6:31–33).

Granted, there is nothing wrong with showing hospitality. But Jesus didn't rebuke Martha for being a gracious hostess. Certainly breaking bread with friends was of the utmost importance. But Jesus didn't correct her for serving her guests. Jesus corrected Martha because she did exactly what He said *not* to do: she worried, and didn't "seek first the kingdom." Martha had tunnel vision. Her fretting left her unable to see beyond her to-do list. The matters at hand distracted her to such an extent that she misplaced her priorities and missed the big picture. Think about it: privileged with a visitation from the Messiah; the God of the universe sitting in her living room. Would it *really matter* if the food got cold?

The problem with worry is that by magnifying the inconsequential, we blind ourselves to what's important. Surely if Jesus is in the house then nothing else matters. The time we spend wringing our hands would be better spent basking in His presence.

TREATING ANXIETY

Ideally, treatment for any health condition is based on the results of scientific studies and clinical trials. Problems arise when the data doesn't adequately represent a particular group. For instance, with heart disease, many of the early clinical trials were biased toward white men. Researchers didn't recruit enough women and minorities to participate. It turns out there are gender and racial differences in the way heart disease manifests in people. There are even differences in the effects medications have on different groups.

A similar problem exists in the mental health arena, where ageism has played a role. We have an abundance of data on how to treat children, adolescents, and young adults with anxiety disorder. Not nearly as much research has been conducted on older adults and the elderly. Thankfully, this trend is changing. More recent studies have ensured that all age groups are fairly represented.

Cognitive behavioral therapy is the gold standard for treating anxiety disorders in children and young adults. It's now being utilized more frequently in older adults and seniors. There are definite advantages to this approach for the latter, particularly with respect to reducing the number of prescription drugs. Behavioral therapy incorporates several approaches, including

- repeated exposure to situations that provoke anxiety;
- curtailing the tendency to avoid or escape the source of anxiety; and
- changing the way of thinking about issues that generate fear.

Like with depression, the combination of behavioral therapy with medications is an acceptable approach. In older men and women, the rule of thumb is to start with a low dose and increase slowly if necessary. This helps to minimize side effects and drug interactions, which can be serious. Benzodiazepines, for instance, are drugs frequently used for anxiety. For older adults, they are often overprescribed or given in too high a dosage. Confusion and instability are two of the more serious side effects, which both increase the chance of falling. And falls, of course, can lead to hip fractures, head injuries, and even death.

I have personal experience with this very issue that could have had disastrous consequences. At this writing, my mother is eighty-four years old and (by God's grace) entirely independent. She recently faced fairly extensive dental work. Considering her lifelong aversion to even walking into a dentist's office, you can imagine how the thought of spending several hours there distressed her. Knowing of her fear, her dentist prescribed a single dose of diazepam (Valium) to take the morning of the procedure. A benzodiazepine, this medication is used for chronic anxiety disorder but is sometimes prescribed for isolated stressful events.

When my sister arrived at Mom's home that morning, my mother was incoherent. Then she became unresponsive and fell down, prompting my sister to call 911. An ambulance took Mom to the emergency room, and a doctor admitted her to the hospital. Thankfully, she did not sustain any fractures or physical injuries. However, what we thought would be an overnight period of observation to allow the drug to clear her system turned into a three-day stay. Her confusion persisted, and the medication caused her heart to beat slowly and irregularly. Even after her discharge, it took a couple weeks before she felt normal. While I knew her dentist had prescribed this drug, I didn't learn until later he prescribed a dose too high for someone her age. Of course, I struggled with feelings of guilt for not confirming the dose beforehand (although still thankful for a good outcome).

Currently, the recommended first-line medications for general anxiety disorder are antidepressants. These were listed in the previous section and are usually well tolerated. But benzodiazepines are in a different category. For most people they are reserved for short-term use, in conjunction with an antidepressant. They include diazepam (Valium), lorazepam (Ativan), and alprazolam (Xanax). Along with the side effects already mentioned, benzodiazepines carry the risk for drug dependence and drug withdrawal.

MENTAL AND PHYSICAL HEALTH

When I wrote *Spiritual Secrets to a Healthy Heart*, I wanted to do a comprehensive examination of the subject. If we consider ways for reducing the risks of heart disease, a healthy diet and exercise come to mind, along with weight loss and kicking the cigarette habit. All play a major role. What we tend to overlook, though, is the mind-body-spirit connection and the way our mental and emotional health impacts the risk for heart disease. So I devoted the entire midsection of the book to this topic.

However, we can't stop with the heart. Nearly every aspect of physical health is influenced by our mental and emotional well-being—heart disease, cancer, diabetes, gastrointestinal diseases, skin conditions, and various forms of arthritis, to name a few. Since chronic illness is more common in older people, this mind-body connection becomes more evident with age. And it's a two-way street: people with medical conditions are at a higher risk for developing depression and anxiety, and mental health disorders will increase the likelihood of developing chronic physical disease. They also increase the risk of death from any cause.

BIBLICAL INSIGHTS

Then they went up out of Egypt, and came to the land of Canaan to Jacob their father. And they told him, saying, "Joseph is still alive, and he is governor over all the land of Egypt." And Jacob's heart stood still, because he did not believe them.
—GENESIS 45:25–26

Jacob's life was packed with high intensity moments. He topped the other patriarchs with respect to ups, downs, and unexpected turns of events. While he likely had some dull periods, much of what is recorded about Jacob in the Book of Genesis could be classified as stressful. One of the more significant episodes occurred toward the end of his life. His favorite son, Joseph, was sold into slavery by his brothers, who fooled Jacob into thinking his son had been devoured by wild beasts. After presenting him with Joseph's bloody tunic (that is, *goat*-bloody tunic), Jacob "tore his clothes, put sackcloth on his waist, and mourned for his son many days" (Gen. 37:34).

Those were tough times for father and son, but God's purpose was greater than the pain. Over the course of years, Joseph's prophetic abilities elevated him from prisoner to powerful government official, and he became one of the most influential leaders in Egypt. In this capacity he encountered his brothers, who went to Egypt looking for food during a famine. When they appealed to Joseph, they had no clue of his identity. In due time Joseph revealed himself, and requested that they tell their father he was alive. This shocking news proved too much for Jacob, who by this time was an old man with an old man's heart. Genesis 45:25–26 records his response and gives an excellent example of the mind-body connection. The *physical* reaction was significant—Jacob's heart actually stopped beating. Stress hormones likely triggered this disturbance in the normal rhythm. After hearing the news, a surge of these chemicals was released into his bloodstream, with a toxic, potentially life-threatening effect on his heart.

The Bible reveals here what medical research now confirms: there is an inextricable link between physical, mental, and emotional health. It is not possible to be whole without appreciating the connection. Those who age gracefully will embrace total wellness—body, mind, and spirit.

Chapter 8

MENTAL HEALTH PART 2: MEMORY AND COGNITIVE FUNCTION

*If it had not been the LORD who was on our side,
when men rose up against us, then they would have
swallowed us alive, when their wrath was kindled
against us; then the waters would have overwhelmed
us, the stream would have gone over our soul; then
the swollen waters would have gone over our soul.*

—PSALM 124:2–5

NOT SURPRISINGLY, MENTAL health is also associated with cognitive and neurological function. Depression in particular is a risk factor for dementia. If left untreated, depression can even mimic dementia. Memory loss, dementia, and loss of cognitive function represent some of the major fears people have about growing older.

Before going any further, though, let me offer a word of encouragement: misplacing your keys is not the same as having Alzheimer's disease! Still, after age forty, it seems forgetfulness—however minor—becomes a source of major concern. I am in no way minimizing the impact of dementia. Right now it is one of the more serious health issues we face as a nation. And for some people, trivial bouts of forgetfulness are the precursor to significant impairment. But even though dementia is common—currently an epidemic—it shouldn't cause us to worry. (Didn't we just talk about worry?) Instead, become proactive by enhancing your lifestyle and improving your overall health. Stick with good habits and get rid of bad ones. Plenty of data supports the essential role a healthy lifestyle plays in lowering the risk for dementia. So going up and down the stairs hunting for your keys is not so bad!

"Normal" aging includes some degree of memory loss. Only about one in one hundred people go through a lifetime with no detectable change in their cognitive function. The vast majority of people experience some decline—most commonly with memory—which can be aggravating, but does not hinder their ability to function. So a spectrum exists extending from the 1 percent who age with no deficits, to those who are partially disabled, and on to those completely incapacitated by dementia. Within this range we find the condition known as "mild cognitive impairment," which has received considerable attention in the media and the medical community in recent years.

MILD COGNITIVE IMPAIRMENT

Mild cognitive impairment (MCI) is fairly common. Its prevalence ranges from 10 percent to 20 percent in people over sixty-five. There are two forms: amnestic and non-amnestic (or, in lay terms, forgetful and not forgetful). Amnestic MCI is memory loss that is significant but not severe enough to meet the criteria for dementia. While sufferers are aware of their deficits (as are their families and friends), their ability to function is fairly well preserved. In the less common form of non-amnestic MCI, cognitive decline appears in areas not related to memory. Problems with language, the ability to maintain focus and complete tasks, and the visual-spatial skills needed for safe driving may suffer.

Many studies have shown people with mild cognitive impairment are at higher risk for developing dementia. Still, making the distinction between normal aging and MCI can prove challenging. Misplacing keys is a nuisance, and forgetting names aggravating, but at what point should a red flag go up? Typically, MCI memory loss is more prominent than that of normal aging. People can't recall things they once easily remembered like meaningful dates (i.e., birthdays and anniversaries) and the content of recent conversations. They also forget things that normally capture their attention. An avid baseball fan who can't remember which team won the most recent World Series may have more than benign forgetfulness.

While it may be tricky to differentiate MCI from normal aging, the distinction between MCI and dementia is usually obvious. With dementia, cognitive deficits have a significant impact on functioning and the ability to live independently. Of course, of major concern for people with MCI (and their families) is whether they will steadily decline, especially since MCI is a risk factor for dementia. And while the condition may indeed worsen, certain factors predict a more rapid progression, including the severity of impairment and whether there is a genetic predisposition.

Currently, no medications are approved for treating MCI. Drugs used for Alzheimer's disease have not shown any benefit in people with MCI because they don't slow the rate of progression to dementia. However, there is some evidence that cognitive rehabilitation—memory association, mnemonics, and intellectually stimulating activities—may help. A doctor should conduct a thorough evaluation for depression, since this can cause memory loss. Lifestyle modification, particularly exercise, also plays a role in improving cognitive function and slowing progression. We will discuss these measures in more detail in the next section.

BIBLICAL INSIGHTS

For what great nation is there that has God so near to it, as the LORD our God is to us, for whatever reason we may call upon Him?... Only take heed to yourself, and diligently keep yourself, lest you forget the things your eyes have seen, and lest they depart from your heart all the days of your life. And teach them to your children and your grandchildren.

—DEUTERONOMY 4:7, 9

Much of the Book of Deuteronomy consists of Moses's farewell speech to the Israelites. It is a heartrending time: they stand on the brink of entering the Promised Land, yet their leader will not be making the journey with them since God denied Moses that privilege. Moses feels anxious about their future, since they are about to enter a land occupied by foreign nations and people who worship false gods. The temptation to turn to idolatry will be tremendous. It doesn't help that Moses knew firsthand how their parents went astray. After all, they were the ones who worshipped a golden calf in the wilderness.

So in his final petition, Moses is passionate about one thing: don't forget God. Over and over again he tells them remembering God represents their highest priority and most important challenge. In this passage he encourages them to continually remind themselves and their children of this. Moses knew the best safeguard against going astray was maintaining a fresh recollection of who God is and what He had done. In doing so, they would never have reason to question the truth that theirs is the one true God. So he pleaded with them to remember, especially the events of the past:

- Don't forget your miraculous escape from Egypt.
- Remember how God protected you in the wilderness.
- Think about the daily provision of manna from heaven.

Tragically, with the fall of mankind, disease entered the world. Our once perfect bodies became imperfect. The long list of imperfections includes memory loss, whether as part of normal aging, mild cognitive impairment, or dementia. In the usual progression, the first thing to go is short-term memory. Consequently, we can recount events of the distant past in great detail, but what happened yesterday escapes our recollection.

I believe this is evidence of God's grace and a manifestation of His kindness. Though memory loss is an aftermath of the Fall, God in His mercy allowed our *distant* memories to be the most resilient.

How does this show evidence of His mercy? Because like the children of Israel, we too should make it a practice to reflect on God's faithfulness. I quoted part of Psalm 124 at the beginning of this chapter; I am especially fond of the phrase that starts verses 1 and 2, "If it had not been the LORD who was on our side..." Then David goes on to remind them of past events and how God showed up just in the nick of time to deliver them. Thank God for long-term memories! They encourage us, revive us, and stir up a fresh devotion to God. Yes, there may come a time when we won't remember what happened a few hours ago. But we will still be able to reminiscence on days long past when the Lord made a way out of no way. There may come a day when we struggle to recall a recent conversation. But we won't have any trouble remembering how God, in yonder years, proved to be a Provider, a Helper, and a Friend. Rejoice in the goodness of God and the blessing of memories.

DEMENTIA

Dementia is an acquired condition. In other words, no one is *born* demented. It develops over time and is characterized by a decline in at least two of the following areas: memory, language, attention, visual-spatial capabilities, and executive function. The last on this list is more difficult to assess than memory or language. Executive function involves such things as the ability to plan, organize, problem solve, make decisions, and think abstractly. The decline must be significant enough to hinder a person's ability to function, either socially or in the workplace. Behavioral changes and psychological symptoms are two other features.

The number of people with dementia is difficult to determine, but for the United States estimates range from 2.5 million to 5.5

million. Of the many risk factors, age is the most significant. The estimated prevalence by age is as follows:

- Ages seventy to seventy-nine: 5 percent

- For those in their eighties: 24 percent

- Over ninety: 37 percent

Racial differences are fairly pronounced and stem from a variety of reasons. About 8 percent of whites over age sixty-five have dementia, compared to about 20 percent of African Americans and Hispanics.[1] Several studies also show a gender disparity, with a higher incidence in women. However, this difference is more likely a reflection of women's longer life expectancy.

Alzheimer's disease is one of several forms of dementia, and also the most common. Because it is so widespread and has received so much attention in recent years as the population ages, it is fairly common to hear the name used erroneously. Irrespective of the cause, people with signs of cognitive decline are often labeled as having "Alzheimer's Disease." However, while various forms of dementia may have identical symptoms, the underlying causes between each differ. Some features of the four most common forms are:

- Alzheimer's disease (60 to 80 percent): the memory loss with Alzheimer's is gradual. In many cases it only becomes apparent after the individual loses a key care provider, often the spouse. Adult children might not appreciate the degree of impairment in one parent until the other parent dies. The deficits will manifest themselves with a change in daily routine, such as relocation. People with Alzheimer's disease may have paranoid delusions or depression. Early on, language and speech deficits may be the most noticeable feature, although personality and neurological function are typically preserved at this point. As the disease progresses, other cognitive deficits become apparent, along with such neurological problems as seizures, tremors, and weakness. Aphasia is common and manifests as a difficulty in finding words ("it's on the tip of my tongue") or stalling midsentence to recall the appropriate word. Multilingual men and women may forget the language they learned most recently, or speak in a mixture of dialects.

- Vascular dementia (10 to 20 percent): this form of dementia is caused by any condition that reduces brain circulation, most commonly following a stroke. A key feature is that function will deteriorate in a "stepwise" manner, becoming more pronounced with each subsequent stroke. Typically, impaired judgment and decision making are more prominent than memory loss, at least initially. This form of dementia should be suspected in anyone with risk factors for cardiovascular disease, even if other typical signs of stroke (like weakness and paralysis, for instance) aren't present.

- Dementia with Lewy bodies (10 to 25 percent): Lewy bodies are abnormal clumps of a specific protein found in the outer portion of the brain. The loss of memory and cognitive function is similar to that of Alzheimer's disease. Individuals with this type of dementia are also prone to hallucinations, delusions, sleep disturbances (nightmares and sleep walking), and muscle rigidity.

- Mixed dementia (10 to 30 percent): this is the term used when more than one form of dementia is present. For example, a person with Alzheimer's may suffer a stroke and also develop vascular dementia.

Keep in mind that memory deficits and behavioral changes can stem from disorders other than these common forms of dementia. So before we go further in our discussion on dementia, let's review a few conditions that can adversely affect memory, behavior, and mental status:

- Delirium. This leads to significant behavioral changes with wide fluctuations in the level of alertness. There can also be agitation, mood swings, and even hallucinations. Making the diagnosis is critical, because delirium is frequently caused by a condition that can be treated. Drug overdose, medication interactions, metabolic problems (low oxygen or low blood sugar, for instance), and organ failure are common causes.

- Depression. Both depression and dementia can cause apathy. But apathy from the latter is typically offset by positive stimulation. A person with dementia will often perk up in the presence of family, friends, food, and fun. Not so with depression.

- Subdural hematoma. This should be suspected in the setting of any head injury or fall. Headaches may be common, as well as fluctuations in the level of consciousness.

- Traumatic brain injury. Like subdural hematoma, this includes a history of head trauma. Symptoms vary according to the part of the brain injured.

- Vitamin B_{12} deficiency. This can lead to a variety of findings, including dementia, depression, nerve damage, and anemia.

- Thyroid disease. Both an overactive and an underactive thyroid gland can cause mood and behavioral changes.

- Brain tumor. As with traumatic brain injury, the clinical findings reflect the location of the tumor. Frontal lobe tumors cause memory loss and cognitive decline.

- Syphilis. When syphilis affects the brain, it leads to a wide range of symptoms, including memory loss, personality changes, delirium, depression, and dementia.

- Alcohol. Long-term alcohol use can cause dementia. This is frequently permanent, but in some cases it will reverse after a period of abstinence.

- Toxins. Exposure to toxins in the form of heavy metals (e.g., lead, arsenic, mercury), aromatic hydrocarbons, solvents, and drugs of abuse (e.g., marijuana, opiates, cocaine) can affect brain function—often permanently.

- Other causes. A number of medical conditions—including multiple sclerosis, systemic lupus erythematosus (SLE), severe liver or kidney disease, and chronic infections—can cause changes in cognition, behavior, and memory function.

MORE ON ALZHEIMER'S

Because Alzheimer's is the most common form of dementia, it is worth covering in greater detail. Like dementia with Lewy bodies, in Alzheimer's proteins accumulate in the brain. This forms "plaques" and "tangles." A protein known as beta-amyloid forms the plaques; the twisted fibers in the tangles are comprised of tau protein. A *definitive* diagnosis requires a brain biopsy to confirm the presence of these lesions. But a diagnosis can be established on clinical findings alone.

The Alzheimer's Association (www.alz.org) has created a list of ten early signs and symptoms of Alzheimer's disease:

1. Memory loss that disrupts daily life

2. Challenges in planning or solving problems

3. Difficulty completing familiar tasks at home, at work, or at leisure

4. Confusion with time or place

5. Trouble understanding visual images and spatial relationships

6. New problems with words in speaking or writing

7. Misplacing things and losing the ability to retrace steps

8. Decreased or poor judgment

9. Withdrawal from work or social activities

10. Changes in mood or personality

Any of these signs—whether in yourself or a family member—warrants a visit to the person's primary health care provider. A full physical and mental health evaluation is part of diagnosing the condition, particularly whether a person has dementia or one of the many other conditions listed in the previous section.

The exact *cause* of Alzheimer's is unknown, but there are several risk factors for developing this disease. Age is an obvious risk—the disease is unusual in people younger than sixty-five but affects nearly half of men and women over eighty-five. Genetics play a key role. Some genes, like apolipoprotein E-e4 (APOE-e4), enhance the risk but do not necessarily mean the disease will develop. Another category of genes is less common, but those who are carriers are certain to develop dementia. Three proteins have been identified in people who are carriers: amyloid precursor protein (APP), presenilin-1 (PS-1) and presenilin-2 (PS-2). This hereditary form is called "autosomal dominant Alzheimer's disease" or "familial Alzheimer's disease." It has an early onset (even as young as ages thirty to forty) and affects several family members in multiple generations.

Indeed, the risk factors of age and genetics are beyond our control—we cannot do a thing to change the year we were born or our DNA. But there is still good news! Some risk factors for Alzheimer's disease are within our capacity to modify. Head trauma, for instance, is a known risk. Some studies show that people who have sustained moderate to severe head injuries are twice as likely to develop Alzheimer's or other forms of dementia. And while we cannot prevent some accidents, we can lower the odds of sustaining a serious head injury through simple measures like using seatbelts, wearing sports and bicycle helmets, and "fall-proofing" our home.

It turns out that attitude may be another modifiable risk factor. The Cardiovascular Risk Factors, Aging, and Dementia Study has followed a group of participants for many years, monitoring several variables—including attitude. In the assessment on cynicism and distrust, participants were asked to agree or disagree with statements such as, "Most people are honest chiefly through a fear of being caught," "I think most people would lie to get ahead," and "Most people will use somewhat unfair reasons to gain profit or advantage rather than lose it." The researchers found that people who scored high in cynical distrust also had a higher risk of dementia compared to those who scored low. So an "attitude adjustment" proves beneficial to the body and the mind.

Additionally, a large volume of research has confirmed a link between a heart-healthy lifestyle and a lowered risk for Alzheimer's and other forms of dementia. It turns out the same measures used for maintaining cardiovascular health also help to preserve a sound mind (once again, the mind-body connection reveals itself). Since there is no known cure for Alzheimer's disease (the current medications only *slow* the progression—they don't *halt* it), it makes good sense to focus on prevention. This issue was addressed at the 2014 meeting of the American Association for Geriatric Psychiatry. At that meeting, Dr. Kristine Yaffe, a professor of psychiatry, neurology, and epidemiology at the University of California San Francisco, presented data on risk factors for dementia. Her research shows that up to half of all cases of Alzheimer's disease are attributable to these seven modifiable risk factors:

- Diabetes
- Smoking
- Midlife hypertension
- Midlife obesity
- Physical inactivity
- Depression
- Low educational attainment

The overlap of dementia risk with heart disease risk is striking. While diet, per se, is not included on the list, it plays a major role in diabetes, hypertension, and obesity. Avoiding processed foods lowers dietary sodium, which in turn reduces blood pressure. And a Mediterranean-type diet, comprised of primarily plant-based foods and low in saturated fat, is protective for both the heart and brain. Interestingly, weight gained during the middle-age years (when many folks start to "pack it on") is particularly risky. We will discuss these issues further in chapter 9.

We can also reduce the chance of developing dementia by keeping our brains stimulated. This explains why low educational attainment is a risk factor. People who challenge their minds while young create a "cognitive reserve," or "brain cushion." The concept is that of a buffer created by keeping the mind actively engaged to build up brain cells and connections. Then, whatever you lose over time (through aging or dementia) will be offset by the "reserve," minimizing the degree of impairment. Of course it's best to start young, but you're never too old to stir up brain cells. Challenge your mind. Stay curious and involved. Make a commitment to lifelong learning. Get involved in such diverse activities as the following:

- Reading and writing

- Crossword or other puzzles (my favorite is Sudoku)

- Attending lectures and plays

- Engaging in stimulating conversation

- Enrolling in courses at your local college or community group

- Playing cards and board games

- Learning a new craft or hobby

- Cooking and gardening

- Practicing memory exercises

BIBLICAL INSIGHTS

And it came to pass, when all the people had completely crossed over the Jordan, that the LORD spoke to Joshua, saying: "Take for yourselves twelve men from the people, one man from every tribe, and command them, saying, 'Take for yourselves twelve stones from here, out of the midst of the Jordan, from the place where the priests' feet stood firm . . . that this may be a sign among you when your children ask in time to come, saying, 'What do these stones mean to you?' Then you shall answer them that the waters of the Jordan were cut off before the ark of the covenant of the LORD; when it crossed over the Jordan, the waters of the Jordan were cut

off. And these stones shall be for a memorial to the
children of Israel forever."
—JOSHUA 4:1–3, 6–7

I find it comforting to know that God doesn't have
an issue with memory prompts! In so many passages
of Scripture He encourages His people to remember,
even advising them to make something—an altar or a
monument—to recognize a meaningful time or event.
Here, God told Joshua to build a memorial out of
twelve stones. But not just any stones. He told Joshua
to select them from the dry bottom of the Jordan riv-
erbed, one stone for each of the twelve tribes. Then
as future generations would recall stories passed down
from their forefathers, they would know it was not a
random collection of rocks. The legacy of God keeping
His promises and miraculously bringing them to the
Promised Land would live on.

Memories are indeed a blessing from God. And it
is always a good idea to take care of God's blessings.
Optimal memory function depends on good nutrition,
regular exercise, and adequate rest. The latter is particularly important; during sleep we consolidate all the
events of today into the memories of tomorrow. Like
our muscles, the brain operates on the "use it or lose
it" principle. So resolve to use it. Stretch your cerebral
capacity to the limits. Exchange passive stimulation for
active engagement. Don't just watch the movie—read
the book! Don't just listen to music—learn to play an
instrument! And by all means, be like Joshua and use
prompts to your advantage. Make a rhyme, create a
visual cue, form an acronym, or set it to music. To this
day I can recite the Preamble of the Constitution of
the United States, decades after my eighth grade exam.
How did I master it? I learned the preamble as a song,
and the melody stuck in my head. How wonderful it is
to maintain the capacity to remember and to reflect on
what the Lord has done—this is a blessing from God
that is worth preserving.

Although research is ongoing, at present there isn't a cure for Alzheimer's dementia. Some medications help slow the progression of memory loss. Other drugs help with specific symptoms such as behavioral changes, agitation, hallucinations, and insomnia. Alzheimer's is the sixth leading cause of death in the United States, claiming the lives of 500,000 seniors each year. For men and women over sixty-five, it is the fifth leading cause.[2] The disease is overwhelming on several fronts, not just medical. It drains the patient, their finances, and their families' emotional and financial reserves. As discussed in chapter 4, the burden on caregivers can be tremendous.

On a final note, there are dozens, even hundreds of clinical trials examining various aspects of Alzheimer's and other forms of dementia. Some studies recruit people who already have symptoms, while others are looking for volunteers with normal brain function or family members of people with Alzheimer's. I would encourage you to investigate what is available in your area. If you are eligible, don't be afraid to participate. Every clinical trial gives the medical community useful information about dementia: how to prevent it, how to treat it, and—hopefully, one day—how to cure it.

Chapter 9

PRESERVING HEALTH AND PREVENTING DISEASE

Beloved, I pray that you may prosper in all things
and be in health, just as your soul prospers.

—3 John 2

W HILE GOOD HEALTH is a blessing at any age, as we grow older, we cherish this blessing on a higher level. The things we took for granted in the days of our youth! Ignorance is bliss indeed! We couldn't conceive of a time when random aches and audible joints would represent the "new normal," not to mention moles popping up overnight. Thankfully most of these changes are more a nuisance than a serious problem. They constitute what we call "normal aging."

Still, not every nuisance is normal. Age brings an increase in the prevalence of disease; chronic diseases are particularly more common in the senior population. Heart disease, stroke, chronic obstructive pulmonary disease (COPD), cancer, type 2 diabetes, dementia, obesity, and arthritis all fall within the category of chronic disease—and they are widespread among Americans. In 2010, medical authorities attributed seven of the top ten causes of death to a chronic disease. At this writing, about half of all US adults have at least one; one in four has two or more.

"Successful survivor" and "usual survivor" are phrases found in medical literature to describe the aging process. Researchers define success using the following four categories:

- No history of diabetes, heart attack, coronary artery bypass surgery, congestive heart failure, kidney failure, stroke, COPD, multiple sclerosis, Parkinson's disease, amyotrophic lateral sclerosis (ALS, often known as Lou Gehrig's Disease) or cancer (excluding more common forms of skin cancer)

- No impairment in cognitive function

- No physical disabilities (not hindered by usual activities; only moderate limitation with more demanding activities)

- No limitations related to mental health

Doctors define successful survivors as men and women who reach age seventy while meeting all four criteria. Usual survivors reach that age with at least one of the four. Clearly, some criteria are not tied to habits and behaviors, but it is also evident that lifestyle plays a major role in whether or not we age with success.

BIBLICAL INSIGHTS

No longer drink only water, but use a little wine for your stomach's sake and your frequent infirmities.
—1 TIMOTHY 5:23

Apparently Timothy, Paul's "son" in ministry, was prone to feeling under the weather. In this scripture Paul gives him advice on how to treat his ailments—use a little wine. A key distinction here is that this would have been wine with medicinal properties, not a drink that would lead to drunkenness. Although we don't know the specifics of Timothy's condition, I pointed out earlier that he had a tough pastoral assignment, particularly from those in his congregation who disrespected him because of his youth. Now since the *physical* symptoms of stress often show up in the digestive track, his stomach problem may have been stress related (it's not clear from the text, but possible).

We also know Paul had no reservation in giving him advice to take something to feel better. If Timothy were alive today, he would likely obtain an over-the-counter remedy or a prescription medication. First, a cautionary note: a healthy lifestyle is always in order. Proper diet, adequate exercise, and minimizing stress go a long way toward keeping us healthy, especially with respect to chronic diseases. However, sometimes this approach is inadequate, meaning a medication is in order. If this describes your situation, just think about Timothy. Set your goal on healthy living, but don't fret if you have to take a pill or two.

Many health commentators use "burden" in describing chronic diseases. What a fitting term. They place a tremendous burden on several fronts—on the individuals, their families, the health care system, and the economy. Chronic diseases are expensive. In 2010 86 percent of all US health care spending originated with people with one or more chronic conditions.[1] They are a leading cause of disability. As an example, almost half of the fifty-three million adults diagnosed with arthritis say it limits their daily activities. And while the average life expectancy has increased, chronic disease offsets those gains when people spend those added years ill and disabled.

So whether we are sick or healthy later in life depends to a great extent on personal choice. For chronic diseases, our risk increases or decreases according to habits and lifestyle. Naturally, some risk factors are beyond our control. Age, race, genetics, and even socioeconomic status all play a role. However, several unhealthy behaviors are within our power to change. The following four are responsible for much of the illness, disability, and premature death related to chronic diseases:

- Improper nutrition

- Inadequate physical activity

- Tobacco use

- Excessive alcohol use

When it comes to chronic disease burden, I have good news and bad news. First, the good: these diseases can often be prevented, or at least their onset can be delayed. The results of many studies show that 10 percent to 50 percent of adults are "successful survivors." Those who reach seventy (and beyond) without a single chronic illnesses and maintain full physical and cognitive function prove the burden is not inescapable. The bad news: the majority of adults are not escaping. On the contrary, too many Americans are caught in the trap of chronic disease, growing old under a burden of often-preventable conditions.

Successful aging—graceful aging—requires embracing a lifestyle that maximizes wellness. Likewise, we reject (or at least minimize) risks that compromise good health. The burden of chronic disease is tremendous, but a healthy lifestyle serves to protect us. Likewise, screening tests and immunizations are useful to detect and prevent many conditions. In this chapter we will cover some of the practical matters that help preserve health and prevent disease.

Keep in mind, while good health is a blessing, graceful aging involves more than personal health status. In a broader sense, graceful aging is a sacrificial commitment—which brings us back to the issue of choice. Aside from the personal pain, the economic burden of chronic disease is tremendous. Simple lifestyle choices influence the cost: what we eat, what we drink, whether we smoke, and how much we move. Our economic burden won't disappear either, with the debt passing on to our loved ones. This is where sacrifice comes into play. We owe it to our children to leave an inheritance of health and prosperity. We owe it to our government to do our part in ensuring a strong economy. Most importantly, we owe it to the Lord. He has given us wisdom to make choices for better health, and He's given us power to stick with those choices. Indeed, God is glorified through a lifestyle of discipline, moderation, and self-control.

NUTRITION AND PHYSICAL ACTIVITY

Diet and exercise are foundational to good health. The risk of major chronic diseases like heart disease, diabetes, and many forms of cancer either increase or decrease according to the quality and quantity of food we eat and our level of physical activity. Additionally, diet and exercise are major determinants of physical capacity. Three of the leading causes of disability—arthritis, obesity, and frailty—are all influenced by how much we eat, what we eat, and whether or not we exercise. While the well-established links to medical conditions are irrefutable, more recent data is confirming that the health effects go beyond physical disease. Nutrition and physical activity even affect mental health and cognitive function.

Aging gracefully is rooted in the simple principle outlined in my book *Spiritual Secrets to Weight Loss: Eat Well; Eat Less; Move More*. Diet plays multiple roles: what we *do* eat, what we *don't* eat, and how *much* we eat all impact our health. The quantity we eat relates to the issue of obesity and being overweight. In the United States, obesity constitutes an epidemic in every age group, but the health consequences become more pronounced over time. It places us at risk for all types of diseases, including chronic conditions of diabetes, cancer, arthritis, and cardiovascular disease. Obesity also predisposes us to a number of non-chronic conditions. Acid reflux, gallstones, and urinary incontinence, for instance, all become more common as body weight goes up.

Food *quantity* plays a role in body weight, but food *quality* is important for overall health. Some foods are beneficial and protect us against disease. The vitamin- and nutrient-rich plant-based foods are good examples. Other foods are detrimental and contribute to disease. Foods and beverages high in sodium, saturated fat, trans fats, sugar, and high fructose corn syrup can heighten the risk for chronic diseases. Ideally, our diets should contain a majority of plant-based foods. For nonvegetarians, low-fat dairy, fish, and poultry are also good choices.

BIBLICAL INSIGHTS

Oh, taste and see that the LORD is good.
—PSALM 34:8

David could surely attest to the grace of God. In Psalm 34, he writes about how God sustained him, protected him, and delivered him from trouble. In verse 8, he uses the imagery of food to convey his pleasure in the Lord. God's goodness and mercy is like a delectable treat. It's delightful!

Israel rests along the Mediterranean Sea. So when David used food to describe the goodness of God, his frame of reference would have been a Mediterranean diet. I think that is fascinating. Why? Because research has consistently shown this type of diet—whose components haven't changed much since David's time—is beneficial to our health. In general, a Mediterranean diet includes the following:

- Lots of vegetables, fruits, and whole grains
- Regular servings of nuts, seeds, and legumes (beans, peas, and lentils)
- Low amounts of red meat and processed meat, with more fish and lean poultry
- A higher proportion of monounsaturated fats than saturated fats

People who eat in this way enjoy better health, aging with more strength and vitality compared to those who follow a standard "Western diet." No doubt, the Lord is concerned with our *total* well-being. The Psalms tell of

how He preserved David in times of trouble and protected him from his enemies. But the Lord also gave
him foods to preserve his health and protect him from
disease. And they delighted his taste buds to boot! We
can experience the benefits of these same foods today.
Surely God preserves and protects us on every front—
O taste and see that He is good!

Back in 1978, Johnny Mathis and Deniece Williams sang a duet
that reached number one on the US Billboard Hot 100 Pop Chart.
"Too Much, Too Little, Too Late" was the hit single from the album
(remember albums?) *You Light Up My Life.* An ironic title for the
album, considering the message behind the hit song: the couple
agreed their relationship offered nothing worth salvaging. So
instead, they sang a pretty song about it. How depressing.

Thankfully, the "too little, too late" principle does not apply to
nutrition. Certainly the benefits of food are maximized by a lifetime of eating well, which is one of the reasons we must teach good
habits to our children. Chronic diseases don't develop overnight,
and the beneficial (or detrimental) effects of dietary components
take many years to show their cumulative effects. However, it is
never too late for change, a fact confirmed by recent data from the
Nurses' Health Study.

The Nurses' Health Study originated in 1976 and enrolled more
than 120,000 female nurses between the ages of thirty and fifty-five.
Participants completed questionnaires at the start and every two
years since. The study has gleaned considerable information, particularly with respect to aging. A recent data analysis involved a subset
of close to 11,000 women who had no chronic diseases back in the
1980's, when they were in their late fifties. These women provided
information on their health status fifteen years later. Researchers
learned that the quality of the diet, even at midlife, continued to
have a significant impact on overall health. The odds of successful

aging increased by about 40 percent in those middle-aged women who maintained a healthy diet.[2]

Irrespective of our years, we are what we eat. Our food choices—both quality and quantity—determine our risk for many chronic conditions. Consider the following diet-disease relationships:

- Sodium: hypertension, heart disease, stroke, kidney failure

- Saturated fat: heart disease, stroke, peripheral vascular disease

- Sugar: weight gain, dental caries, inflammation

- Calories: obesity with its long list of consequences, including diabetes and arthritis

The potential for harm is clear. We must also factor in the other side of the coin, namely the health benefits found in nutrient-rich foods we Americans so commonly leave off our plates. The vitamins, minerals, phytonutrients, and antioxidants found in natural foods work to lower our risk for chronic diseases. Nor can you just replace good food with a pill. In general, we reap the benefits of these nutrients when we consume them from *dietary* sources, not supplements.

In 2014, after an exhaustive review of solid evidence gathered from clinical studies, the US Preventive Services Task Force updated their recommendations on this issue. The guidelines apply to a specific group of people: healthy adults without nutritional needs. Certainly, there are some individuals who need to use nutritional supplements. So the advice of the USPSTF does not apply to children, people with known nutritional deficiencies, those who are chronically ill or hospitalized, pregnant women, or women attempting to get pregnant. But for otherwise healthy adults, there are no advantages to using vitamin, mineral, and multivitamin supplements for disease prevention. The health benefits come from consuming the actual foods, rather than isolated nutrients that have been synthesized and placed in pill form. And this makes sense, even biblically. In Genesis God ordained the fruit of the earth to sustain us—not pills from a bottle.

Indeed, a good diet is vital to aging gracefully; so is physical activity. The effect of exercise is similar to that of diet for the odds of being a successful survivor—the benefits are not limited by age. The Nurses' Health Study evaluated this in a subset of nearly fourteen thousand women. All were free of any chronic diseases at the start, and all survived to at least age seventy. Investigators found a strong link between midlife physical activity (whether structured exercise time or active leisure time) and health status in later years. Not surprisingly, women with higher levels of physical activity had a lower incidence of chronic disease, fewer disabling conditions, and were less likely to experience limitations from mental health disorders. And, they were more likely to maintain full cognitive function. The really good news is the benefits were apparent, irrespective of body weight. So in both lean and overweight women, those who moved more aged better.[3]

As for how much physical activity is recommended, I encourage you to visit the Centers for Disease Control and Prevention's website (www.cdc.gov/physicalactivity) for detailed and helpful information. For adults, the general guidelines are as follows:

- One hundred fifty minutes of moderate-intensity aerobic activity PLUS at least two days of muscle-strengthening activity every week

OR

- Seventy-five minutes of vigorous-intensity aerobic activity PLUS at least two days of muscle-strengthening activity every week.

Bear in mind, these are the *minimum* amounts recommended for *preserving* good health. In many circumstances, including weight loss and diabetes control, more activity will yield better results. In general, higher levels of exercise bring greater benefits, provided you don't push yourself to the point of injury. Along with setting aside time for working out, it's also important to be more active in daily life. Look for opportunities to move. So stand when you can, walk if the distance is reasonable, and take the stairs instead of the elevator.

Finally, remember chronic diseases become more common as we age, and in their early stages they may be silent. If you have risk factors for heart disease, get a medical evaluation before embarking on an exercise program, even if you're feeling well.

TOBACCO AND ALCOHOL

Nicotine is highly addictive, which explains why smoking is still common despite the known health risks. More than forty-two million US adults are smokers; this habit accounts for more than 480,000 deaths annually.[4] Tobacco use and secondhand smoke increase the risk for chronic diseases, particularly heart disease, COPD, and many forms of cancer. The good news is that you're never too old to quit. Smoking cessation significantly reduces the risk of death from chronic disease, even for longtime smokers.

Quitting is not easy, but it is possible. Some succeed in going "cold turkey," but others need a little more help. Behavioral counseling is useful. There are several medications with proven effectiveness, including bupropion (Zyban), varenicline (Chantix), and nicotine replacement therapy. Relapses are common, so don't let this discourage you. Just get back on track and summon the determination to kick the habit.

Drinking too much is another major cause of preventable disease, with about 88,000 deaths each year attributable to alcohol. Alcohol-related problems stem from both acute intoxication and the long-term effects. Accidents and injuries are examples of the former, while organ damage and cancer are examples of its chronic toxicity. Unlike tobacco, where no level of consumption is safe, light alcohol consumption is generally safe and has only minimal health risks. There are obvious exceptions when abstinence is best, including during pregnancy, or if a person has a past history of alcohol dependency or other forms of substance abuse.

BIBLICAL INSIGHTS

Who has woe? Who has sorrow? Who has contentions? Who has complaints? Who has wounds without cause? Who has redness of eyes? Those who linger long at the wine, those who go in search of mixed wine.
—PROVERBS 23:29–30

Heart disease is the number-one killer in America, and its prevalence increases with age. Naturally, people who are aware of this tend to look for ways to lower their risk. Diet and exercise are mainstays, but there is considerable data showing benefits of light to moderate alcohol consumption. So, then, should a person start drinking for a healthy heart? Probably not, mainly because the risks of alcohol easily outweigh any health benefits.

Proverbs summarizes well the injury, sadness, and broken relationships of alcoholics—"those who go in search" for a drink. Along with the social consequences and the potential for addiction, excessive alcohol use carries serious health risks. For the sake of clarity, "moderate" drinking is up to one drink per day for women and up to two for men. For women, "heavy" drinking is defined as having more than three drinks on any given day, or more than seven drinks during a week's time. Heavy drinking for men is having more than four drinks on any given day, or more than fourteen per week. What constitutes a "drink?" A standard drink contains fourteen grams of alcohol. Generally, this amount is found in:

- 12 ounces of beer;
- 8 ounces of malt liquor;
- 5 ounces of wine; or
- 1.5 ounces (a "shot") of 80-proof liquor.

Excessive alcohol can damage several of the body's organs, especially the brain, liver, and heart. Moderate to heavy drinking also increases the risk for many types of cancer including breast, liver, colon, rectal, esophageal, and those involving the head and neck. Clearly, these risks outweigh the cardiovascular benefit. So here's the bottom line, at least in my book: if you don't drink, don't start. There are plenty of other ways to protect yourself against heart disease. If you do drink, keep it light. And if drinking is a problem, seek help to overcome that, and then permanently abstain from alcohol.

IMMUNIZATIONS

Vaccines are not just for children. But since adults don't deal with expulsion from school, it is easy for our "shots" to lapse. The Centers for Disease Control and Prevention have recommended the following immunizations for adults, based on age and medical condition:

Recommended Adult Immunization Schedule—United States - 2015

Note: These recommendations must be read with the footnotes that follow containing number of doses, intervals between doses, and other important information.

Figure 1. Recommended adult immunization schedule, by vaccine and age group

VACCINE ▼ AGE GROUP ▶	19-21 years	22-26 years	27-49 years	50-59 years	60-64 years	≥ 65 years
Influenza[*]	1 dose annually					
Tetanus, diphtheria, pertussis (Td/Tdap)[*]	Substitute 1-time dose of Tdap for Td booster; then boost with Td every 10 yrs					
Varicella[*]	2 doses					
Human papillomavirus (HPV) Female[*]	3 doses					
Human papillomavirus (HPV) Male[*]	3 doses					
Zoster					1 dose	
Measles, mumps, rubella (MMR)[*]	1 or 2 doses					
Pneumococcal 13-valent conjugate (PCV13)[*]					1-time dose	
Pneumococcal polysaccharide (PPSV23)		1 or 2 doses				1 dose
Meningococcal[*]	1 or more doses					
Hepatitis A[*]	2 doses					
Hepatitis B[*]	3 doses					
Haemophilus influenzae type b (Hib)[*]	1 or 3 doses					

[*] Covered by the Vaccine Injury Compensation Program

Legend:

- For all persons in this category who meet the age requirements and who lack documentation of vaccination or have no evidence of previous infection; zoster vaccine recommended regardless of prior episode of zoster
- Recommended if some other risk factor is present (e.g., on the basis of medical, occupational, lifestyle, or other indication)
- No recommendation

Report all clinically significant postvaccination reactions to the Vaccine Adverse Event Reporting System (VAERS). Reporting forms and instructions on filing a VAERS report are available at www.vaers.hhs.gov or by telephone, 800-822-7967.

Information on how to file a Vaccine Injury Compensation Program claim is available at www.hrsa.gov/vaccinecompensation or by telephone, 800-338-2382. To file a claim for vaccine injury, contact the U.S. Court of Federal Claims, 717 Madison Place, N.W., Washington, D.C. 20005; telephone, 202-357-6400.

Additional information about the vaccines in this schedule, extent of available data, and contraindications for vaccination is also available at www.cdc.gov/vaccines or from the CDC-INFO Contact Center at 800-CDC-INFO (800-232-4636) in English and Spanish, 8:00 a.m. - 8:00 p.m. Eastern Time, Monday - Friday, excluding holidays.

Use of trade names and commercial sources is for identification only and does not imply endorsement by the U.S. Department of Health and Human Services.

The recommendations in this schedule were approved by the Centers for Disease Control and Prevention's (CDC) Advisory Committee on Immunization Practices (ACIP), the American Academy of Family Physicians (AAFP), the America College of Physicians (ACP), American College of Obstetricians and Gynecologists (ACOG) and American College of Nurse-Midwives (ACNM).

These guidelines were most recently updated in 2015. The biggest change compared to the prior recommendations is that all adults sixty-five and older should receive two pneumococcal (pneumonia) vaccines: the thirteen-valent pneumococcal conjugate vaccine (Prevnar 13) and the twenty-three-valent pneumococcal polysaccharide vaccine (Pneumovax 23).

Vaccine recommendations differ in the face of certain medical conditions like heart, lung, or liver disease, diabetes, kidney failure, and HIV infection. There are also specific recommendations for people who work in health care. Talk to your health care provider to determine which vaccines are appropriate for you.

Screening

I can imagine if our efforts to stay well were part of a sporting event (the Olympic Games, for instance), the judges would award a gold medal for the previously discussed "Disease Prevention." Proper nutrition ("proper" meaning quality *and* quantity), adequate physical activity, avoiding unhealthy habits, and staying up to date with immunizations are key preventive measures. They safeguard our bodies and our minds and keep us in optimal health. Remember the old saying is true: an ounce of prevention *is* worth a pound of cure.

If prevention captures the gold, then screening would have to get the silver. Ideally we would like to age as successful survivors, with no chronic diseases. However, if we are afflicted, the next best thing is for an early diagnosis of the condition, before it's had a chance to do us much harm. This is the rationale for screening. While such measures do not *prevent* disease, they do afford the benefits of early detection.

BIBLICAL INSIGHTS

Is anyone among you sick? Let him call for the elders of the church, and let them pray over him, anointing him with oil in the name of the Lord.

—James 5:14

Even though I'm a rather ordinary, down-to-earth person, some folks find me interesting. They are fascinated by my faith—specifically my stance on science and faith. I completely embrace both. For me, belief in one does not preclude the other. To the contrary, they affirm one another. I have come to learn this stance is not typical.

However, it is biblical. In this passage, for instance, James addresses the need for prayer in times of sickness. Notice that the verse alludes to prayer and conventional medicine being complementary. We see here a balance of faith and science: yes, bring the oils with medicinal properties, but don't forsake prayer.

In addition, notice that the person with the affliction is expected to be proactive. He or she is the one who is to initiate contact with church leaders. If we aren't careful, sickness can foster self-pity and can even lead to apathy. But there is never a time for passivity. Those who cope best with illness are the ones who take the bull by the horn, so to speak, and maintain an active role in their treatment. And that treatment includes prayer.

In recent years, research in the area of faith and medicine has confirmed the benefits of healing prayer. Secular institutions have conducted studies whose results confound the investigators. However, you can't refute hard evidence; the data speaks for itself. I am not intrigued by the results of such research. I didn't need a clinical trial to prove that prayer works. I am a scientist, but I'm also a woman of faith. God said to pray, and that's enough for me!

Before reviewing some common screening tests, I need to clarify a few basics about screening:

- First, *not every disease has a screening test.* I cannot tell you the number of times I've had patients come into the office wanting to be "checked for everything."

- Second, *not every person is eligible for every test.* The makings of a good screening test merge the disciplines of medicine, pathology, statistics, epidemiology, and economics, along with risk-to-benefit ratios. These are used to determine who stands to benefit from a particular screening. What many non-clinical people fail to recognize is that inappropriate screening is not harmless; it carries potential risks.

- Third, *screening guidelines are dynamic, not stagnant.* Because knowledge, technology, and treatment options change over time, so do the guidelines. A standard protocol a decade ago may not apply today.

- Finally, *screening is intended for people who are symptom free.* If there are any suspicious signs or symptoms, the testing is no longer considered screening; it is performed as part of the diagnosis. For example, if a woman feels a lump in her breast and her doctor orders a mammogram, it is not for the purpose of *screening.* Her mammogram (and likely other tests) will be to reach a *diagnosis.* While this may seem like a lesson in semantics, it makes a huge difference with regard to the type of test ordered, along with proper documentation and insurance reimbursement.

The following list includes a few conditions that are suitable for screening. As always, consult with your health care provider to determine which tests are right for you.

- *Hypertension,* also known as high blood pressure, meets the criteria for a condition suitable for screening. It is common, has no symptoms, and is easily treated. Left undetected, it is a major contributor to illness, disability, and death. In addition, checking blood pressure is convenient, painless, and inexpensive. Screening is recommended for all adults, at least every other year.

- *Diabetes:* In the initial stages type 2 diabetes may not cause symptoms, or feature easily ignored symptoms. And this phase might last for years. Unfortunately, complications of the disease begin to develop during this time. All adults with heart disease, hypertension, or high cholesterol should be screened for diabetes. It is also recommended that adults who have risk factors for diabetes get screened at least every three years. Risks include obesity, a family history of diabetes, age, and being part of an ethnic minority. For women, polycystic ovaries and diabetes during pregnancy (gestational diabetes) are also risk factors.

- *Hyperlipidemia:* Cholesterol screening is recommended for men over age thirty-five and women over age forty-five.

- *Osteoporosis.* Screening is recommended for men and women, depending on age and risk factors. Refer to chapter 3 for more details.

- *Hepatitis C:* In the United States hepatitis C virus is the most common blood-borne infection and a major public health concern. About 2.7 million people are infected, but the majority—as many as 75 percent—are unaware.[5] Left untreated, the consequences of chronic HCV infection include cirrhosis and liver cancer. Current guidelines recommend a one-time screening for adults born between 1945 and 1965.

- *HIV:* The US Preventive Services Task Force recommends screening for HIV as part of routine medical care up to age sixty-five.

- *Cancer:* Some forms of cancer are suitable for screening, while others are not. Various tests can detect breast, colon, cervical, lung, skin, and prostate cancer, whether through a physical exam, blood tests, stool tests, or radiographic imaging. More invasive screening procedures include the Pap smear and colonoscopy. Experts often disagree on appropriate tests, and professional organizations may issue conflicting recommendations. To further complicate matters, screening technology is rapidly evolving. So recommendations are subject to controversy and modified fairly often. Discuss with your health care provider which tests are right for you.

- *Other conditions:* Various tests and tools are available to screen for depression, aortic aneurysm, glaucoma, thyroid disease, alcoholism, and other conditions. Check with your health care provider to determine what is appropriate.

Urinary Incontinence

For many women, loss of bladder control is a debilitating problem that significantly affects their quality of life. A source of embarrassment and discomfort, it interrupts sleep and can limit one's social activities. Yet all too often women don't mention it to their doctor, either because of embarrassment or because they consider it too common a problem to discuss. Instead of seeking treatment, they wear protective undergarments and find the location of the nearest restroom whenever they go out. Yet doctors estimate some form of urinary incontinence occurs in

- Twenty-five percent of women aged fourteen to twenty-one;

- Forty-four to 57 percent of middle-aged and post-menopausal women; and

- Seventy-five percent of women age seventy-five and older.[6]

The most common forms are urge incontinence and stress incontinence. Some women have both, which is called mixed incontinence. With urge incontinence, there is an intense, overwhelming need to urinate followed by the involuntary loss of urine. In stress incontinence, leakage occurs when the abdominal pressure increases—for instance, with coughing, laughing, or sneezing. Risk factors include pregnancy, vaginal deliveries (especially if traumatic), urinary tract infection, cognitive impairment, physical disabilities, constipation, and obesity. Women who have had a hysterectomy or have any condition that leads to a persistent cough are also at risk. The changes that occur in the bladder and urethra with menopause don't necessarily *cause* incontinence, but they predispose a woman to developing it.

With all the pharmaceutical ads for bladder control on TV and in magazines, one would think taking medications is the only treatment option. However, drugs are *not* recommended as first-line therapy; they are reserved for when other measures fail. Losing weight, limiting caffeine, and taking extra bathroom breaks are all helpful, especially for stress incontinence. Some women have a misconception about the amount of water they need to drink. So they consume an arbitrary number of "glasses a day" without factoring in water contained in other beverages and in foods. In case of excessive liquid consumption, just cutting back often does the trick.

Pelvic floor exercises (Kegel exercises) are the recommended first-line treatment for stress incontinence. This involves tightening the pelvic muscles periodically during the day, the same muscles used if you stopped the urine flow midstream. Women who do these exercises properly and consistently notice a significant improvement in bladder control. The key words here are "properly" and "consistently," because Kegel's are easily forgotten during the course of a busy day.

Bladder training is useful with urge incontinence. This is a form of behavioral therapy that requires a woman to create a voiding schedule. The first step is to determine how long you can comfortably stay dry, then make a bathroom-break schedule based on that interval. Next, gradually extend the interval between voiding by about ten to fifteen minutes each week. These measures help improve the bladder's muscle tone and capacity. Rather than rushing to the bathroom, it is also a good idea to take a few deep breaths, sit down, and cross the legs at the first sensation of urgency. These relaxation techniques will allow the initial intense urge to subside long enough to get to the bathroom dry.

Only take medications for bladder control if conservative measures fail. They have several significant side effects. The most troubling are dry mouth, constipation, and blurred vision. If lifestyle approaches and medications fail, other measures are available, including surgery, nerve stimulation, and botulinum toxin injections. Most importantly, don't be ashamed to discuss the problem with your health care provider.

SKIN AND HAIR

I suppose a book on aging wouldn't be complete without a word on skin and hair. Ironically, it's also the last word. Heretofore, I have not focused heavily on outward appearance. Although important, it is an exhaustive topic covered well in hundreds of books and other resources. Even the Bible has something to say about the cosmetics of aging: "Charm is deceitful and beauty is passing, but a woman who fears the LORD, she shall be praised" (Prov. 31:30). Without question, the bulk of our "beauty time" should be devoted to the inside. A beautiful heart is more striking than a flawless complexion. However, for the sake of completeness, I want to review a few points about hair and skin (just be mindful to maintain the right priorities).

BIBLICAL INSIGHTS

The glory of young men is their strength, and the splendor of old men is their gray head.

—Proverbs 20:29

I remember when my first gray hairs started popping up. I wore my hair really short back then, which made them all the more noticeable. There was a crop at my right temple, but nothing on the left. That meant they made my head look asymmetrical, kind of off balance. Who can explain the changes of aging!

Soon after, people started asking me if I was going to color my hair to hide the gray. When I said no, some speculated my decision stemmed from some religious or spiritual reason. A few even referenced Proverbs 20:29; maybe I was glorifying God by preserving my splendid gray head? Not! It wasn't that profound, but represented a personal decision—nothing more, nothing less. I have a lot more gray hair now, and for me it remains a personal choice.

Aging brings about several changes, many that can be modified. Some opt to "age with assistance," while others want each year of their life made evident. Neither approach is wrong or right, just different. Whichever camp you choose, try not to get on a soapbox about it. Learn to respect the decisions of those who do otherwise.

Hair loss is a normal part of aging. About half of the population experiences some degree of thinning by age fifty. Some men start losing hair as early as their teen years. Women are more likely to notice it later, sometimes not until menopause. There is a huge genetic component with respect to the degree and the pattern—whether it begins at the crown or hairline. So if your parents are thinning or balding, chances are you will follow suit.

Yet not all hair loss is normal. Before attributing it to age, make sure you have pursued other possible causes, such as the following:

- Diseases and illnesses: thyroid disorders, autoimmune diseases, chronic illnesses

- Infection: skin infections affecting the scalp, systemic infections, high fever

- Medication: hair loss is a common side effect of many drugs

- Stress: intense stress can cause significant shedding

- Hair styling: chemicals, heat, and excessive traction can lead to hair loss, sometimes permanent

In many ways, hair is similar to skin, reflecting conditions on the outside and the inside. Harsh shampoos, excessive styling, and prolonged exposure to sunlight can damage the hair and strip it of its natural oils, making it dry and brittle. Likewise, the condition of hair is influenced by the quality of the diet and overall health. Barring a few exceptions, hair texture is determined by genetics, so learn to love your DNA rather than fight it. Two exceptions are gray hair and the hair that grows back after chemotherapy. Both have different textures than native hair. The former is more stiff and wiry; the latter tends to be softer and thinner.

Aging affects every part of the body. Skin is no exception. If you examined it under a microscope, you would see age-related changes in the epidermis and dermis, with a progressive loss in the number of cells, blood vessels, and the matrix that holds things together. These changes cause the skin to become thin and delicate. It wrinkles, is less elastic, and is easily damaged by even minor trauma.

The ultraviolet (UV) radiation from sunlight has a similar effect on the skin as aging. Sun damage is referred to as "photoaging." Both time and the sun cause the skin to become lax, with a diminished blood supply. But there are some differences worth noting. Photoaging leads to dryness, deep wrinkling, a leathery texture, and irregular, blotchy pigmentation. However, chronological aging does not cause the same type of pigment changes. And wrinkling is fine, rather than the deep furrows seen with sun damage.

Both chronological aging and photoaging are associated with new growths on the skin. With chronological aging, these are usually harmless. Seborrheic keratosis and angiomas are two of the common, benign, age-related skin changes. They are more of a nuisance than a serious health problem. Not so with the growths triggered by UV radiation, which are often premalignant or malignant.

While we can't turn back the clock on chronological skin changes, prevention is a wise approach for minimizing UV damage. In addition, there are medications and procedures that help to offset the effects of both chronological and photoaging. Here we will discuss prevention and medication. The procedures are beyond the scope of our discussion. They include botulinum toxin, soft tissue fillers, chemical peels, microdermabrasion, and laser technology.

Sunscreen, sun protective clothing, and sun avoidance reduce the damaging effects of ultraviolet radiation—both the cosmetic changes and risks for developing skin cancer. Although melanin is protective, everyone—irrespective of skin tone—should use sunscreen. Choose one with an SPF of fifteen or higher. Apply it liberally to all sun-exposed skin, especially the face, every two to three hours.

Wide-brimmed hats help block the sun too. Clothing is helpful, provided the fabric is actually blocking rays. A loosely crocheted bathing suit cover-up is not going to provide as much protection as a tightly woven fabric. Special sun-protective fabrics have been designed that provide an SPF of thirty or higher. These are especially useful for people who work outdoors, when reapplying sunscreen may be cumbersome.

Obviously, avoiding the sun is a highly effective form of

protection. Ultraviolet radiation is most intense at midday, so try to schedule outdoor activities early, or later in the day. While outdoors, look for shady areas under trees or umbrellas. And finally, sunbathing and sun tanning beds are not advisable, even if you use sunscreen.

Back in the 1980s, researchers found topical tretinoin improved the signs of photoaging. In early studies, researchers found that wrinkles, pigment changes, and the skin's overall texture improved within a year of starting therapy. Tretinoins are currently available in prescription and over-the-counter forms. Although some people develop skin irritation with their use, they are generally safe and can be used indefinitely.

Cosmetics is a huge, multibillion-dollar industry with new products continually appearing. The list of ingredients is exhaustive and includes antioxidants, peptides, and botanicals. These are incorporated into all types of products, from cleansers to moisturizers to makeup. In general, these products appear to be safe, but keep in mind they are not subjected to the same rigorous testing required for the approval of medications. What's more, there are very few large, well-designed clinical trials to confirm efficacy and safety. Since most of the studies are sponsored by manufacturers, bias becomes a serious problem in analyzing the results. It is hard to review data objectively when a concurrent financial investment is at stake. And because regulations are not as strict compared to medications, marketing and advertising campaigns are allowed to make claims based on little evidence. So in all things, practice being a discerning, educated consumer.

BIBLICAL INSIGHTS

All flesh is grass, and all its loveliness is like the flower of the field. The grass withers, the flower fades, because the breath of the LORD blows upon it; surely the people are grass. The grass withers, the flower fades, but the word of our God stands forever.
—ISAIAH 40:6–8

Facials, tretinoin, chemical peels, microdermabrasion—the list of options for enhancing the skin keeps on growing. What we have today would make Ponce de León green with envy. Though on a quest for the Fountain of Youth, this fifteenth- and sixteenth-century explorer (and discoverer of Florida) wasn't the first with that dream. The pursuit to reverse aging started as early as the fifth century BC with the Greek historian Herodotus. Even now we're still searching for ways to look young.

I suppose there's nothing wrong with that, as long as we keep a proper perspective. Indeed a fine line exists between sensibility and absurdity. Using cosmetics to enhance natural beauty is sensible. But in my opinion, surgically generated taut skin on a ninety-year-old face approaches the absurd. Graceful aging means we accept how God created us. We will fade away; He is everlasting. He made us temporal, while He is *timeless*. So why fight it? Accept His sovereignty, and enjoy the ride.

AFTERWORD

Remember your Creator before the silver cord is
loosed, or the golden bowl is broken, or the pitcher
shattered at the fountain, or the wheel broken at
the well. Then the dust will return to the earth as it
was, and the spirit will return to God who gave it.

—ECCLESIASTES 12:6–7

T RANSITIONS SET THE foundation of life. Indeed, they are the essence of the life cycle—not just for mankind but for every living thing. All nature is in the process of change.

Our voyage begins at conception and ends with death. Although a linear path for the individual, in the larger scheme it is part of a cycle. As one life ends, another begins.

Irrespective of our age, each day we live becomes part of our unique journey. It is a forward progression, the rate of which does not change. What *does* change is our perception and our response.

We welcome the transitions of youth. Remember the excitement of the first day of school? Think back on how thrilled you felt to finally receive your driver's license. Or the milestones of graduating, getting married, or purchasing your first home. All delightful moments. Transitions led the way to positive changes, such as independence and self-sufficiency. They ushered in new beginnings. Transitions were the source of joy.

Then something changed. And it wasn't the rate or rhythm of life, which are fixed variables. What changed was the nature of the transitions—and how we reacted to what they represent. Consider menopause, the empty nest, and retirement. Typical midlife changes, but for many, reaching these milestones is not a source of joy. The thrill is gone, replaced by poignant reflections, nostalgia, and even sorrow. Instead of sensing open doors and fresh opportunities, we can reach the painful awareness that the end is closer than the beginning.

While midlife changes speak to the brevity of life, that shouldn't get us down. On the contrary, when you heed Solomon's advice to "remember your Creator," then midlife and late life become times of joy and contentment. Rather than remind us of the end, these transitions should compel us to get things right—right now! Lighten up and laugh; be generous to the extreme; learn to say "I'm sorry"; practice saying "I love you" more often. Now, more than ever, don't sweat the small stuff (and to quote the end of the title of the best-selling book, "and it's all small stuff").

Graceful aging means we face each day with a spirit of hope and thanksgiving. I pray that you embrace the moment, and be glad.

—Kara Davis, MD
www.DrKaraDavis.com

NOTES

INTRODUCTION
FIGHTING THE CLOCK

1.   "Sixty-Five Plus in the United States," US Census Bureau, October 31, 2011, http://www.census.gov/population/socdemo/statbriefs/agebrief .html (accessed August 7, 2015).

CHAPTER 1
ADVANCE CARE PLANNING

1.   "Worktable 309: Deaths by Place of Death, Age, Race, and Sex: United States, 2005," Centers for Disease Control and Prevention, April 8, 2010, http://www.cdc.gov/nchs/data/dvs/Mortfinal2005_worktable_309.pdf (accessed August 7, 2015).

CHAPTER 2
ATTITUDES AND EMOTIONS

1.   J. A. Singh et al., "Pessimistic Explanatory Style: A Psychological Risk Factor for Poor Pain and Functional Outcomes Two Years After Knee Replacement," *Journal of Bone and Joint Surgery* (Britain) 92, no. 6 (June 2010): 799–806.

2.   K. H. Pitkala et al., "Positive Life Orientation as a Predictor of 10-Year Outcome in an Aged Population," *Journal of Clinical Epidemiology* 57, no. 4 (April 2004): 409-414.

CHAPTER 3
BONES AND MUSCLES

1.   Virginia A. Moyer, "Vitamin D and Calcium Supplementation to Prevent Fractures in Adults: US Preventive Services Task Force Recommendation Statement," *Annals of Internal Medicine* 158, no. 9 (2013): 691–696.

2.   Ibid.

3.   Heidi D. Nelson et al., "Screening for Osteoporosis: An Update for the US Preventive Services Task Force," *Annals of Internal Medicine*, 153, no. 2 (2010): 99–111.

4.   L. P. et al., "Frailty in Older Adults: Evidence for a Phenotype," *The Journals of Gerontology, Series A, Biological Sciences and Medical*

Sciences 56, no. 3 (March 2001): M146–M156, http://www.ncbi.nlm.nih.gov/pubmed/11253156 (accessed August 10, 2015).

5.   S. Mathias, U. S. Nayak, and B. Isaacs, "Balance in Elderly Patients: The 'Get-Up and Go' Test," *Archives of Physical Medicine and Rehabilitation* 67, no. 6 (June 1986): 387–389.

CHAPTER 4
COMMUNITY AND SOCIAL NETWORKS

1.   Shan P. Tsai et al., "Age at Retirement and Long-Term Survival of an Industrial Population: Prospective Cohort Study," *British Medical Journal* 331, no. 7523 (October 2005): 995, http://www.bmj.com/content/331/7523/995 (accessed August 10, 2015).

2.   Frank Newport, "Americans' Church Attendance Inches Up in 2010," Gallup Poll, June 25, 2010, http://www.gallup.com/poll/141044/Americans-Church-Attendance-Inches-2010.aspx (accessed August 10, 2015).

3.   A. M. White et al., "Social Support and Self-Reported Health Status of Older Adults in the United States," *American Journal of Public Health* 99, no. 10 (October 2009): 1872–1878.

4.   Cheryl E. Woodson, *To Survive Caregiving* (West Conshohocken, PA: Infinity Publishing, 2007), v.

5.   R. D. Adelman et al., "Caregiver Burden: A Clinical Review" *Journal of the American Medical Association* 311, no. 10 (2014): 1052–1060.

6.   S. M. Parks and K. D. Novielli. "A Practical Guide to Caring for Caregivers," *American Family Physician 2000* 62, no. 12 (December 15, 2000): 2613–2620.

7.   Mathy D. Mezey, *The Encyclopedia of Elder Care* (New York: Springer Publishing Company, 2001), s.v. "caregiver burden," 112.

CHAPTER 5
INTIMACY

1.   "Sexuality at Midlife and Beyond, 2004 Update of Attitudes and Behaviors," American Association of Retired Persons Research, 2005, http://www.aarp.org/research/topics/life/info-2014/2004_sexuality.html (accessed August 10, 2015).

2.   A. Nicolosi et al., "Sexual Behavior and Sexual Dysfunctions after Age 40: The Global Study of Sexual Attitudes and Behaviors," *Urology* 64, no. 5 (November 2004): 991–997.

3.   Jacques Baillargeon et al., "Trends in Androgen Prescribing in the United States, 2001 to 2011," *Journal of the American Medical Association Internal Medicine* 173, no. 15 (2013): 1465–1466, http://archinte.jamanetwork.com/article.aspx?articleid=1691925 (accessed August 10, 2015).

4.   G. Gandaglia et al., "Risk of Myocardial Infarction in Patients Receiving Testosterone Therapy: Still a Matter of Debate," *Annals of Pharmacotherapy* 48, no. 12 (December 2014): 1665–1666.

5.   A. Morales, "Erectile Dysfunction: An Overview," *Clinics in Geriatric Medicine* 19, no. 3 (August 2003): 529–538, http://www.geriatric.the clinics.com/article/S0749-0690%2802%2900104-0/abstract (accessed August 10, 2015).

6.   J. S. Brown et al., "Urologic Complications of Diabetes," *Diabetes Care* 28 (2005): 177–185.

CHAPTER 6
Loss, Control and Hope

1.   William B. Yeats, *The Oxford Book of English Verse*, ed. Christopher Ricks (Oxford, England: Oxford University Press, 1999), 525.

2.   "Statistics Quotes," BrainyQuote, http://www.brainyquote.com /quotes/keywords/statistics.html (accessed June 17, 2015).

CHAPTER 7
Mental Health Part 1: Depression and Anxiety

1.   David S. Brody et al., "Identifying Patients With Depression in the Primary Care Setting: A More Efficient Method," *Archives of Internal Medicine* 158, no. 22 (1998): 2469–2475, http://archinte.jamanetwork.com/article .aspx?articleid=1105615 (accessed August 10, 2015).

2.   Kurt Kroenke, Robert L. Spitzer, and Janet B. W. Williams, "The PHQ-9: Validity of a Brief Depression Severity Measure," *Journal of General Internal Medicine* 16, no. 9 (September 2001): 606–613, http://link.springer .com/article/10.1046/j.1525-1497.2001.016009606.x (accessed August 10, 2015).

3.   N. M. Simon et al., "Informing the Symptom Profile of Complicated Grief," *Depression and Anxiety* 28, no. 2 (February 2011): 118–126.

CHAPTER 8
Mental Health Part 2: Memory and Cognitive Function

1.   *African-Americans and Alzheimer's Disease: The Silent Epidemic,* Alzheimer's Association, 2003, https://www.alz.org/national/documents /report_africanamericanssilentepidemic.pdf (accessed August 10, 2015).

2.   Melonie Heron, "Deaths: Leading Causes for 2010," National Vital Statistics Reports, 62, no. 6, http://www.cdc.gov/nchs/data/nvsr/nvsr62 /nvsr62_06.pdf (accessed August 10, 2015).

CHAPTER 9
PRESERVING HEALTH AND PREVENTING DISEASE

1. "Chronic Disease Overview: The Leading Causes of Death and Disability in the United States," Centers for Disease Control and Prevention, May 18, 2015, http://www.cdc.gov/chronicdisease/overview/index.htm (accessed August 10, 2015).

2. Cécilia Samieri et al., "The Association Between Dietary Patterns at Midlife and Health in Aging: An Observational Study," *Annals of Internal Medicine* 159, no. 9 (2013): 584–591, http://annals.org/article.aspx?articleid=1763229 (accessed August 10, 2015).

3. Qi Sun et al., "Physical Activity at Midlife in Relation to Successful Survival in Women at Age 70 Years or Older," *Archives of Internal Medicine* 170, no. 2 (2010): 194–201, http://archinte.jamanetwork.com/article.aspx?articleid=415545 (accessed August 10, 2015).

4. "Tobacco-Related Mortality," Centers for Disease Control and Prevention, February 6, 2014, http://www.cdc.gov/tobacco/data_statistics/fact_sheets/health_effects/tobacco_related_mortality/index.htm (accessed August 8, 2015).

5. C. M. Wray and A. M. Davis, "Screening for Hepatitis C," *Journal of the American Medical Association* 313, no. 18 (2015): 1855–1856.

6. A. Qaseem et. al., "Nonsurgical Management of Urinary Incontinence in Women: A Clinical Practice Guideline From the America College of Physicians," *Annals of Internal Medicine* 161, no. 6 (2014): 429–440.

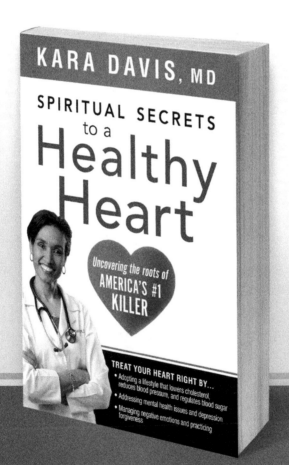